The CARAVAN

of

LOVE

Reporting on The HIV/AIDS Epidemic

DONALD SHARPE

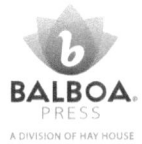

BALBOA.
PRESS
A DIVISION OF HAY HOUSE

Balboa Press books may be ordered through booksellers or by contacting:

Balboa Press
A Division of Hay House
1663 Liberty Drive
Bloomington, IN 47403
www.balboapress.com
1-(877) 407-4847

Because of the dynamic nature of the Internet, any web addresses or links contained in this book may have changed since publication and may no longer be valid. The views expressed in this work are solely those of the author and do not necessarily reflect the views of the publisher, and the publisher hereby disclaims any responsibility for them.

The author of this book does not dispense medical advice or prescribe the use of any technique as a form of treatment for physical, emotional, or medical problems without the advice of a physician, either directly or indirectly. The intent of the author is only to offer information of a general nature to help you in your quest for emotional and spiritual well-being. In the event you use any of the information in this book for yourself, which is your constitutional right, the author and the publisher assume no responsibility for your actions.

Any people depicted in stock imagery provided by Thinkstock are models, and such images are being used for illustrative purposes only. Certain stock imagery © Thinkstock.

Printed in the United States of America.

ISBN: 978-1-4525-7796-8 (sc)
ISBN: 978-1-4525-7798-2 (hc)
ISBN: 978-1-4525-7797-5 (e)

Library of Congress Control Number: 2013912616

Balboa Press rev. date: 7/22/2013

Acknowledgements

Ed and Sunny I thank you for seeing me for who I am. Your kindness will never be forgotten. Lisa Nelson you traveled with me on this journey to South Africa and I am thankful to you for doing so. It was a delight traveling together. My brother Derrick you were scared but you encourage me to fulfill my dream. My wife Bovene you corrected my sentence structures, encourage me to take some rest and to continue to work hard. To my parents, Edna Campbell, Judith, Chevonese, Marsha, sist. Grant, sist. Dozz, sist. Barbara, bro. Wollery, Delroy, Jadon, Jonathan, Nadeen all friends and family thank you for your encouragements. Tom Smith, you were the Executive Nursing Supervisor at Mt. Sinai Hospital who gave me a financial gift I used to purchase a computer I used to document my journey on The Caravan of Love; thank you for taking the time to listen to me before I went to South Africa. Doctor Yogesh Kumar, you are my private doctor for many years. When I told you I was going to South Africa, you made sure I got all the necessary medications I needed to take. You too are a fighter against HIV/AIDS; continue to care for your patients.

"Advance Praise"

"When I read about your trip to South Africa, I was amazed and encouraged. You went to experience what you read about. I hope many more will be bold to bring comfort to those in need. Continue on this journey; be passionate about what you fighting for." Barbara.

"The moment you shared with me and allowed me to read your work on your trip to South Africa, I was astounded. Your work is not just about a crisis, it allows people to have a sense of hope when face with impossibilities in this life. I am a newly graduated teach, I recommend this book for all to read" Chevonese.

"This is a well written book. I am not saying this because the author is my husband. I am encourage knowing that people of all back ground can read this book and find themselves mystified and seeking to do more good for others. Sometimes we forget who we are until some unintended crisis comes our way. This book encourages us to be alert and caring for those who are less fortunate than ourselves. The HIV/AIDS disease cannot be ignored. This is one issue we cannot sweep under the carpet." Bovene F

"I am a nurse. When I read your work, I was encouraged and I encouraged you to share your work with others. Your work took a personal look at the battle many faced, fighting this disease. I encourage parents to get a copy of this book and share it with their children. HIV/AIDS is a disease we cannot afford to ignore." Judith

INTRODUCTION

Caravan of Love
My Trip to South Africa

I HAVE NOW ARRIVED at a place in my life where I know the truth; for years I have tried to ignore it. It wasn't long ago before I realize the truth; I hope it does not take you as long to come to this conclusion. I have finally realized that we all had similar difficulties getting a full grasp of the facts, that life can be unpredictable. No one knows this better than me. Life has some demanding questions, when not answered honestly, sometimes leads us to our own destructions. I encourage you to be courageous, honest and truthful to yourself as well as to others, regardless of the outcome. The phrase, putting your pass behind, is easier said than done. Although we believed we have moved on, memories of our past, sometimes take us back, making us hostages of our past.

Despite each day, each moment that has gone by, unseen challenges sometimes engulf our present; bring us back to moments better left forgotten. We can all look ahead and imagine where we want to go; while memories of our past keeps us looking back at where we come from. No doubt the mysteries of life have plenty of lessons to be learned from. Despite dismal outlooks, there are lessons in life we all have to experience. We all have to learn to forgive ourselves. Remember; share what life's lessons teach you with others, so awareness can be made through your experience.

On this journey you will be encouraged to be awaken to life's lessons in this world we live in. You will read about people suffering from the HIV/AIDS epidemic; do not be frighten or judgmental. We will get started by informing and educate the public about this disease. Despite of all the set back, we will arrive at the darn of a new beginning. Here new supporters will be called to action; there are so many ways we all can contribute and be helpful to someone suffering with this disease. Sometimes we forget to do the easiest gestures to someone in need; just saying a simple good morning or hello. Our aim is to look for better tomorrows; regardless of how good or bad yesterday may have been, I believe it the human dream within all of us to look for a better future. Leaders may have failed to come to a full grasp of the impacts people are going through, because of neglect of facts or ignorance. Despite their failure, we will not stop until the truth about our suffering is realized. With such a disease, you do not have to be infected to be affected. In fighting this disease around the world, we need to eliminate barriers to testing and treatments of this disease. There need to be more assertive measures taken to help reduce rape: raping of young girls for the sole purpose of ridding yourself of this virus. Many are loosing their hold on assaulting young girls as sex slaves because the world is crying foul while these girls of gained a measure of pride within themselves; they have answered the call to action. This can ensure and help encourage children to seek ways for a better tomorrow. It is wonderful to see adults help children develop strategies to support themselves regardless of the obstacles they may face. Yes, some adults teach the young people in their communities how to prepare for tomorrow by teaching them to cultivate crops for the market place. You will read about starting a new beginning. This includes forgiving yourself of mistakes of the past and starting over with a new hope, driven with passions to live.

A few days ago I woke up with the sun shining down on my face through a thin lace curtain I had over the bedroom windows in my apartment. Awaken by the sun shining on my face from a restful night sleep, was to me a gracious awakening greeting me and welcoming me into the spark of a new day. It is nice to wake up just to enjoy the splendor of a new day. I took my time getting up, knowing I had fully used up all the time I needed for a good night's rest. Now I am prepared to face the new day with a bright outlook. I would not allow this moment to escape me without showing my appreciation and thankfulness; not everyone goes to sleep and wakes up with such vigor to face the new day ahead. When you have a purpose or a mission to accomplish in life it makes a big difference getting up and starting your day right. There are no guarantees that your day will go the way you want it to, instead, we might have to learn to make some adjustments to what lies ahead. We need to remember to place emphasis on important things in life, such as having good health, good food to eat, a place to rest, and a better future for ourselves, our children and family. There are defining characteristics that one look for to identify if they are living a prosperous life. It can be the availability of medical services whether far or near, but it must be available or the access to work so someone can make a better life. This may not be a lot for many people around different parts of the globe, because this is all that they got. But for those people awaken in sickness without access to a medical facility, it can be devastating. Awaken and not have money to provide food on the table is wrenching to the hearts of many people. These people may feel alone and that no one cares for them. They may feel abandoned by their own communities because it seems everyone is going through something similar. Despite feeling alone and abandoned, it does not have to be like this. I assured you, with humans' compassion and generosities we will over come from life's darkest moments as we work together to overcome some of life's impossibilities.

Take for example a few nights ago I was walking home on a long stretch outside to my apartment. What I noticed amazed me. When all appeared to have gone to their bed, the breeze of the night was the only movements I felt whispering in my ears. It made me walk faster, but the faster I walked the more I felt the arms of the breeze cuddling me. Looking around I saw nothing, only when I looked up I saw something that amazes me; the moon in the sky was shining down at me. My fear went away and I was comforted to know that a light was shining down at me. There was no one there, but the presence of that light made me feel safer knowing it makes it easier for someone to recognized and identify my presence if I had to make a loud cry.

Have you ever stop for a moment and think why everywhere you go the sun or the moon always follows you? No matter how fast you walk or even run, they often seem to be right there over your head. As adults we often do not asked these questions, but as a child growing up I did. As a little boy I used to run as fast as I could, trying to find a hiding place where I could escape from the sun or moon. I am often disappointed, because no matter how fast I ran, the sun and moon are always there following me. I am not the only one to question these events. Flocks of birds often fly in a group, trying to out fly the sun. They too probably have asked the same question I have asked, can we ever out fly the sun? The answer is no. There is one thing I do admire about flocks of bird flying together, despite a lonely few often got left behind; they often make that clocking sound. I believe this is a signal, indicating where and which direction they are heading. This is there way of texting each other. At the end of their desired destination, all will be accounted for. They may not all reach at the same time, but a strong bird would be there to guide the weaker ones.

As human beings, we often miss out on so many little things; we are so busy with the cares of life that oftentimes quiet moments for great appreciation passed us by unknowingly. I am here to let you know that we are always covered by a great force of energy or light and it is up to us to stop for a moment and realized this. It does not matter what you are going through in life or trying to run away from, you are not alone. Yes there are some moments when clouds will appear and block the sun or moon light so the place may look dark but clouds cannot remain around or over us for ever. They have to empty their heavy loads that will eventually wet someone below, or water the ground for growth of fruits and vegetable, for fishes of the sea to swim in and grow; so we all can have something to eat. You see no matter what dark clouds comes our way; we have to ride it out on our caravan. Whether we travel by day or night, there is always a guiding light that is there to help us through. The moon and sun are not always fully lit. If you listen to the weather report from time to time you will hear phrases such as partly cloudy or partly sunny. I just found out recently that partly cloudy means there will be more sun than clouds and partly sunny means there will be more clouds than sun. Sometimes the moon is quarter, half or fully lit. We need to have in our caravan something to help us see ahead if the elements will be partly cloudy, partly sunny, a quarter or half moon. What will be found in your caravan? Could it be a torch, a flash light, a pin light, love or emptiness?

Sometimes we need a little help to forge ahead. Sometime we cannot see the light around us, but it is there. The greater elements above never stop shining. When one stops the other picks up. Sometimes we may need to obtain something to see through a dark tunnel, but I guarantee you it won't be long before you will see the beauty of the heavenly lights. We may need to wait awhile before we can move on if you do not have some way of seeing ahead. We are never alone. Yes you may not be able to see ahead, but someone will come along and help us to realize that hope and peace is ahead. This journey you will take with me is about that, joining together not feeling left alone. It does not matter if we are walking alone at night or traveling in a busy crowd during the day, we need to know that we are not alone. There is someone next to us that can help us through this journey.

Chapter 1

AWAKEN

NOT OFTEN DO YOU open a book and discovered what the ending of that book will be within the first couple of pages, or the author tells you what the book is about within the first page. That will happen with this book you are about to read. Despite finding out what the ending of this book is about early in the book, it will be one of the most exciting books you have ever read. Why is the author doing this? There must be something going on that he is unable to control. Not so! We read to discover things about people, places or events, but there comes a time when we need to learn something about ourselves. This book calls for the human spirit to go beyond the surface of what has been said, and look for the real intention of our existence, why we are the way we are, what makes you different from someone else, questioning why some people are more fortunate than others, it makes you asked the question where am I on this path of life and finally what can I do to make this world a better place?

That happened to me when I read a news paper article on HIV/Aids. That is why I am doing the same thing to you. Discovering what a book is about within the first page, does make that reading seems uninteresting. We live with ourselves each day and sometime it takes years to discover things about our own selves. Sometimes it is difficult for us to believe or even understand the different dimensions of our lives and existence. In this book you will experience romance, hate, love, despair, abandonment, abuse, rejection, mist trust, deceit, knowledge deficits, disappointment, hopelessness, hope, fear of the unknown, anger, faith, loneliness. Most of all, you will discover yourself. This book is more about people discovering who they are and finding ways to come to an understanding about their existence in a way that brightens the life of another person.

The conclusion of this book is about you. I have never met you, but I can predict that despite all you read about this book, it does not end at the last page. The ending of this book is the beginning of what you will do to make a difference in the world around you. Don't feel alone; it's now a few years later since 2001, when I first read the article on HIV/AIDS in South Africa and I am still doing something about this journey I am on. I do not have a time limit set for when I should take an exit; knowing myself, making an exit might just lead me back to the same path or to something similar. Make the end of this book as interesting as can be; your story will encourage someone to change their way of thinking. Enlighten someone to make discoveries. Empower someone to take a stand despite whatever difficulties they are going through. It will allow someone to embrace themselves and start over with a new beginning. Most of all, someone who has been diagnosed with this deadly disease may find assurance and peace of mind reading this book. When all appears to be lost, life has a unique way of rejuvenating itself. As life tries its best to make a new beginning, we too should not loose hope. Instead, let this be a new beginning for a brighter future. Now I feel free; the pressure is off me making a lousy ending to this book. Remember now, the ending you make will have an impact on generation to come. You will have your time to think about it and may even share it with the world.

In a small way you and I are connected and we will remain connected throughout this journey, which I have called, "The Caravan of Love." Love helps us to share the common good of all; love has no weight, no stagnation. We all have an empty part within us which I call the caravan. Before motor vehicles were created, carts were created with wheels pulled by mules, donkeys or horses; these were called caravans. Caravans were used to carry loads from one point to the next. On this journey you will travel in my BMW; best made wagon.

The caravan has no color, no shape, no length, no width and no depth. However, the more we fill our caravan with good things, the bigger it gets. It's a part of us we all share. Some people learn or discovered how to make their caravan work better or faster for the up-liftmen of others. What you fill your caravan with is up to you. My caravan is filled with love ignited by a force greater than any force known to man. I refused to let this journey end even if tested along the way; let's turn to each other not against one another. I became aware of my caravan when I read an article written about HIV/Aids in South Africa. I do not believe that I am different from anyone else. I believe you can learn something about yourself by looking into your caravan. We are living in a time where we all need to be involved in taking care of the world we live in; no more procrastinating!

It was a slow morning from what I can remember; I was at work. In the interest of helping the day go a little faster, I started to straighten up my work area and refill supplies I would need throughout the day. I can remember the calmness of that morning. No day remain calm in my work setting for too long. Before this calmness disappears, I usually make sure that all additional equipments are in placed. My job involves thinking ahead of all events and listening to those around me. I must make sure that what was not done by the previous shift is taken care of. I make sure that the beds are clean and in functioning order. At each bedside their must be a bedpan or a urinal; in case of an emergent need for an escape from the bladder or bowel. Sometime we all take for granted some of the simple things in life, until there is emergent needs that arise. I realized that this morning when I bought the morning papers before getting in to work.

Later that day when I had a chance to read that news paper article, I have not been the same from that day. What I experienced while reading this news paper article, have made me into a warrior. Had someone called my name while I was reading this paper, I doubt I would have heard them. Yet I was there, but my mind was far away. To get a full understanding of what I read, I remembered reading that article over and over on my break. All I remembered wanting to do, was to get home and read this article all over again. I know you are thinking what this article could be about. No it was not about asking for money. I must tell you that this news paper article was an eye opener for me.

As a way of getting the public enticed to purchase their papers, news paper companies always placed an interesting subject on the cover page. For me it was more than captivating. This one news paper cover page changed my life. We are living on the same earth, but unless something out of the ordinary happens to us, we all continue to live in our own little world. Some of our world involves making more money; others include advancing their status in life through whatever means they decide. Nothing is wrong with that, however, there comes a time when we all have to stop and open our eyes. Failing to see ourselves and the world around us do brings about torments and unhappiness. I am not saying that this is why people may feel depressed, I am just happy that I did not mist out on my calling. There is a two Way Street to one's calling; first the person must answer then he or she must make a loud cry that will echo so far away, this cry will encourage others to come and help.

I have answered my calling, and now I am making a loud cry writing this book. Pay close attention to yourself as you read this book; you may discover your calling. We are living in a world that is too silent while so much of us are living in torments. Some of us do not realize that we are all connected in one way or the other; it is for you to find out how. We have what it takes to make a better world for our today and for our children's tomorrow. When we take a close look at all the discoveries to life's enhancements, most of them have been discovered years ago. The fact is that we won't be around forever, but actions we take can represent us along with motivating other in our generation to greater achievements.

There is something in all of us waiting to be discovered. We do not all have the same enthusiasm or discovery spirits, but something is there waiting to be discovered. When one does not work on their discovery, others left unenthused about life itself. This one young lady wrote about the desperate cry for help because of the HIV/AIDS epidemic in South Africa. I have always wanted to go to Africa; where in Africa I had no idea. However, after reading this article, I am driven to discover this land so far away with so many cry for help. I knew right away that this was my calling. South Africa was thousands of miles away; however, if this article can be so invigorating, then writing this book is something I can do for the world to see.

We were created to achieve or to pursue life's greatest achievement; doing good towards our fellow man. When we all do something good and try to understand each other, no doubt good things follow us. If we should fall short of that expectation, no doubt the God of heaven will be there to guide us and ease our pain and anguish. The anguish of life's torments or claims on human sufferings must come to an end or pause for awhile so children can escape from a world of torture and feel free to live. A break such as this one can allow people of good nature to continue the call of helping those that are in need. As humans we are not perfect, yet call to a perfect mission; one involving making our fellow man happier. This should be an aim for all, especially for the young children. Children should not have to endure this passage of pain and endless suffering. Instead, we should be and are responsible for making an oasis of peace, love, education and compassion for each other. We know that children retain whatever they are taught from an early age. Exposing a child to painful experiences will only make that child believe that it is acceptable to live like this. This belief defeats the human instinct to search deeper within one's self for the quest for optimism and self exploration. This is the twenty first century; we can all learn something from our past. Human optimism can never be taken away or for granted. Through fighting or communicating with one another, we will find a way to pass the mantle of human optimism on.

We need each other to survive from day to day. There is no doubt that there will be a tomorrow; you may not see it, but someone else will. Therefore, for the human spirit of not surrendering and keeping optimism alive, let's get together on the caravan of love. It's not like a plane ride where a reservation is needed or a bus ride where a ticket is needed, not even like a taxi ride where a fare is needed. This is something where we all can participate by being active in caring for one another. On this caravan of love, all we need are each other. We all have emptiness within us, which I call a caravan. A caravan is a space equips to carry load. The strength of your caravan depends on your motivation to overcome life's ups and down. Ironically, someone who had a difficult time through life tends to make their caravan smaller. The less carrying capacity means my pain will be limited also. I know what you are saying, how can that be true? It appears that bad people have far more different arrays of bad things to do. To explain that, it appears so, but that is not true. The fact is, it does not take a lot of bad things to make life difficult; only one. On the other hand, so much love is needed we need to have a bigger carrying capacity of love and goodness to meet the needs of people out there. What you fill your caravan up with is up to you.

My caravan is filled with love; ignited by a news paper article I came across. I read in this news paper article about children, women, families, and communities suffering from the HIV/AIDS epidemic in South Africa. This story was so overwhelming to me; I could not get over it. Although it was so heart wrenching, I read it over and over. I did this looking for an answer I could not find. I keep asking my self, why? But no one was there to give me an answer. So I open myself to understand what was going on. I share this story with you now. This will be an opportunity to find where you fit in and maybe discover your caravan. World leaders are needed to enforce laws and make decisions for a better future; however, their roles are not like ours. We are more powerful than all world leaders. We all need to take a stand and embrace change for a better tomorrow; no more procrastination. I remembered reading that news paper articlet; on the front page was an interesting article on the outbreak of HIV/AIDS in South Africa. I became enticed to read this article. I cannot explain why at the time, but now I know. I was about to be called on a mission, a mission of love. I read this article about children suffering because their parents were dying. Hospital and staff members exhausted and frustrated because there seems to be no end to the dying of young people ages twenties to forties, and the suffering of young children. The government of South Africa was lost to what was happening, while the word stood by hoping that their own eyes would open to what was going on when it comes to HIV/AIDS. Now as a health care worker myself, I could understand the frustration and confusion that was going on. I could not understand the helplessness a developed nation would allow its people to undergo surrounds this one issue involving the HIV/AIDS crisis.

I was confused and did not know what to do. I remembered screaming, asking myself what I can do to help. I asked myself why the reporter wrote this article. What was she trying to accomplish? Was she trying to get help for these people suffering, even though she did not ask for help? Am I going beyond myself trying to help with such a world crisis? Why someone would write an article like this, expecting nothing in return? She gave all the detail about her research, yet she asked for nothing. Am I going beyond myself trying to do something when nothing is expected of me? Well, I had something else planned. I wanted to know what I could do. Maybe this article was only published for customers to purchase more of this news paper. If this was the case I would purchase more news paper article; an inquirer mine like mine always like to know more about what is happening. For me this was more. One's destiny comes along quietly, only for you not to be distracted by what is going on around you.

After reading this article, my main question was what can I do? And who could I speak with to help me to do something? Well, it did not take me long. I called the news paper itself, the following day. I called up the news paper; it was the New York Times. The person who answered the phone was very helpful. Up to this day I cannot forget how helpful and understanding the person who answered the phone was. I thought that they would have given me the run around; collecting my telephone and name then maybe call me back. It was not so; instead I got the telephone number of the reporter in South Africa right away.

I hurried home the night before going to bed to read this news paper article; tonight again I hurried home to make a very important call. I kept that telephone number in a safe place where it would not be lost. Of course I could call the news paper again for the telephone number of the reporter. However, I kept that telephone like a map to a hidden treasure. When I got home I went to sleep right away to get up at midnight eastern time to make a call to South Africa. Fortunately I have a prepaid phone card, one I used to call my wife who was living abroad. Using a prepaid phone card is less expensive than to use my phone directly to make a call half way across the world. With my excitement to call South Africa, I forgot to find out the time zone; how many hours ahead they were from us. Despite my over zealousness, I made the call at midnight. The first good thing was that they were eight hours ahead of us; so someone was probably awake to answer my call.

I did not know what to expect calling someone who wrote an article like the one I read. I was not a person donating money to assist in improving or assisting in the suffering this community was going through with the spread of HIV/AIDS crisis. I was just calling to find out what I could do in helping this community. In my wild thinking, maybe she had people called her before and put her on a wild chase wasting her time. I did not know what to expect. In my little self, I called and waited in anxiety as the phone rings. Finally, someone answers the phone; it was a male, the reporter's husband. I introduced myself as a nurse who read an article written by his wife that was recently published in the New York Times. He was very friendly and sounded happy that someone was responding to an article written by his wife. He told me that his wife was not available at the moment, but he would give her the message and that I could call back another time to speak with her.

The next time I decided to call South Africa was on my day off. Staying up after midnight and going to work later that day was not easy on the body. From the short time I spoke with the reporter's husband, I learned a few things. First I learned that they were eight hours ahead of us. This was helpful in helping me to plan my next call carefully or I should say timely. Speaking with the reporter's husband was very helpful. Before I tell you what happen with the next phone call I made, I must introduce you to this wonderful inspiring writer; her name is Rachael Swarns. I must tell you that I was very lucky to have Rachael picked up the phone the next time I called; it was as if she was waiting for my call. I introduced myself to her as a reader of the news paper article she wrote on the crisis with HIV/AIDS in this small town in South Africa named Hlabisa. She sounded excited right away. She told me a little about her work in South Africa as a journalist. One of the things she discussed with me was the fact that she was limited with getting a whole lot done, but she could introduce me to people who could help me. One particular person she told me about was a young medical doctor who is very helpful in showing her around, his name is doctor Hlengwa. I cannot forget, she understood that making a call between these two countries was expensive, so she mentioned that this phone call was probably expensive and we should communicate by email. We exchanged email addresses and said goodbye to each other; this was in November 2001.

Words cannot explain the way I felt after talking with Rachael. This was more than just a simple phone call; to me it was a dream come through. I felt very comfortable talking with her. She made me feel wanted; this inner feeling empower me to feel that I have what it takes to accomplish what I set my mind to do. Talking to her helped pushed me towards accomplishing this mission. Hope without bearing fruit is very painful. I have been rescued, and with this opportunity I will bring about hope to those who are giving up on life. A few weeks ago here in NYC, terrorist demolished two famous buildings and killed many innocent people. I myself had a mission to accomplish, and nothing will stand in my way. Talking to this journalist has encouraged me to look deep within myself for something the world would come to embrace. We lived in a world where it seems as if evil abound. However, within me love flourished for those less fortune, for the weak, innocent children, the elderly, and those who lack knowledge. I will do whatever it takes to spread hope and optimism in the presence of those who are giving up.

Chapter 2

GETTING STARTED

I CHECKED MY EMAIL daily looking for a response from over sea. I was a little disappointed whenever I saw that I did not get an email from South Africa. I was thinking like a little child the day before their birthday on the excitement that lies ahead. I guest; I was thinking what could be taking her so long after getting over my little zealousness; I waited until I got an email from her. I made two copies of the email; one for my personal file and the other to carry around with me reading. It was one thing reading about all the issues this community was having, but now I was making myself responsible for doing something to help.

The first email I got from Rachael, she was able to give a contact person. His name is doctor Hlengwa. She gave me a telephone number to contact him and also his email address. I did not contact him immediately. I called Rachael back a second time. These were the only two times I spoke with her while she was in South Africa. I called her to get a sense of what she felt was needed in these communities. I want to have a little background knowledge on the communities and also I did not want to make commitments to thinks I could not accomplish in a timely manner. I believe helping young children, helping community leaders in educating the community, providing some medical supplies and just being there as a support person for communities going through rough times. I did not want to talk with my contact person with a blank piece of paper. I know that I have some limitation; but I believe that whatever way I needed to assist in this crisis, is possible. One thing I know for sure is that hope not bearing fruits is painful. I did not want to give an impression that I can do it all. I just know that I had to do something within my scope of living.

I called Rachael a second time and asked what she felt were thinks the communities needed. I wanted to have a sense of some of the thinks I could provide. I read about hospital short of supply, and children in need, the community has so much despair, people clinging to sooth Sayers rather than doctor. The entire community/country is in total disarray. These communities need to see something positive happening. Especially the children, they are absorbing so much of this negativity.

We all question ourselves sometimes about what we are doing about a particular task at hand; I did. I began to feel as if I was stepping into the role of the united nation. As fellow humans, we should not allow the people of one nation to under go so much unnecessary pressure. The world community should not come together only when there is a need for war or economic down falls. I believe we can do even better, standing up for people suffering from HIV/AIDS. This medical crisis is affecting and will affect generation to come. In the mean time, people are suffering right now. This was the dilemma I got caught up in; I did not want to do too little or ignoring established governmental agencies nationally and internationally. I was scared not knowing the right thing to do.

One thing kept me going was the fact that I did not start pursuing this endeavor because I heard about it from someone else; I read about it myself and want to do something about it. This is one of the greatest convictions I have ever had. To believe in something that seems so far away, while at the same time so near, I believe will bring out the best in me. I believe in the human optimism to bring about positive changes; a mission to help those in need. We have to remember that progress does not unfold passively; we have to take a stand. In this case, we have to participate in the caravan of love which will over stretch many barriers and smooth the minds of the fainted hearts. Hope of brighter beginnings begins with us. We cannot afford to wait for another generation to take up this responsibility. This is what I am asking of you, I encourage you to journey with me on this trip. I hope that this will be a life learning experience for us. There is so much to learn in life; we cannot procrastinate. It seems sometimes that bad things happen more often than good things. However, that is not true. You and I are proof that although bad things do happen, evil cannot stand against the power of good people. We are resilient, we do not accept short comes and go on with life. We take stands that people around the world can take a look at; and do make similar lifestyle changes.

I started out by collecting pennies or one cent in small jars and as they full up I purred them into bigger containers. I collected them in clear plastic bottles to help me see how far I was moving up each day. I tell you that it was very painful, but I continue to collect my pennies. I started to collect them for two reasons. The first is that I hope to find someone some day that would match every penny I have collected maybe with (10.00, 50.00, 100.00, 500.00, 1000.00 etc with no limits). The second reason was to help set aside money for my trip to South Africa. I prayed, I never gave up hope on myself not being able to go through with this journey. It was not easy; but something was inside of me inspiring me to never give up. I read the news paper article in November of 2001 about the devastation the HIV/AIDS crisis was making in South Africa.

Approximately two years later from the time I read the news paper article on the HIV/AIDS epidemic in South Africa I had a patient at work that fell in love with me. Well, I must be honest; I too fell in love with her too. She is a Caucasian female that came into the hospital for medical treatment for symptoms she was feeling, but after being thoroughly checked out was sent home with a clean bill of health. Before she went home, we got to know each other on a personal level. From day one in nursing school we were all told not to allow your patient to get to know you on a personal level; however for the first time, I did not abide by that rule. I will call her Sunny. I found Sunny to be a very detailed person. She asked questions that the doctors could not ignored about her health. She also was very loving to her husband. I will call him Ed. She worried about him dearly. From what I understood at the time, they had a business together. She tried as much as she could to help her husband run their business while she was in the hospital. After observing Sunny for sometime, I asked her what type of business she and her husband was involved in. She told me. She also let me know that with this business her husband traveled all over the world. I happened to ask her if this included Africa. She said yes. Now, let talk for a minute you and I. Can you imagine where this conversation may go? I do not want you to guest; I will tell you. It will go to the caravan of love. I asked her where in Africa they do business. She told me. After Sunny did most of the talking, I decided to do some myself. I shared with Sunny the news paper article I read on the devastation people was going through with the HIV/AIDS crisis in South Africa.

After sharing with her how I felt and what I planned to do about it, we both fell in love with each other. She told me that she would like to keep in touch with me. From there we exchanged contact information and vowed never to loose contact with each other. You see, Sunny fell in love with me because of the kind and gentle person she got to meet. Sunny was sent home without treatment, because all the symptoms that brought her to the hospital had subsided. The only treatment she needed was to hear about my story which one day may become history. In my mind, we were meant to meet this way. I will share some of the things that I have shared with Sunny that I did not share with you. Since I read the news paper article I have been a warrior. I have collected ventilators from my hospital and have sent them over to South Africa. I have also rented a van and collected old computers from my hospital to be sent over to South Africa.

I did not kept what I read in the news paper article to myself. Almost everyone knew my story. I was at work when one of the material coordinator, Patricia came up to me and told me that the hospital had bought some new ventilators and was dumping out the old ones. I was happy to hear this bit of information. I had to work fast. I need to find a shipping company that ships things to South Africa. I started to search all over the place. I almost gave up until I found one in Brooklyn, NY. After getting some detailed information about cost, delivery port and tariff rates, I decided to go with them. I had to arrange a fast pick up of the two ventilators at the hospital.

I thank Patricia who was the material coordinator at Mount Sinai

Hospital. She helped me arrange the pick up of the ventilators from the hospital. Nothing can leave the hospital without the necessary clearance. Out of her busy schedule, she arranged help for me to assist me in getting the ventilators outside the hospital. I used my own transportation to do the pick ups and to take them to the shipping company. The ventilators were inspected. At first when I called the shipping company, I told the owner what I was sending, and the reasons why I was. I told him I was sending the ventilators to my friend to be delivered to the Hlabisa Hospital who is in need of much medical equipment. Something very strange happened on the day I went to the shipping company. I must tell you that the owner was an African American male. After my two ventilators was inspected by him, I saw a man walked into the store started talking to the manager then both of them started to inspect the ventilators. I asked him why this man was looking at the ventilators. He told me the man was looking to see if he could help sponsor the shipments. I prayed that these ventilators would arrive to South Africa and some day I would see them working helping to save the lives of someone. I must be honest, ever since that day, I never see or heard about them. They were to be delivered to doctor Hlengwa who was to take them to the Hlabisa Hospital. I had no doubt that this was an arrangement set up by the shipping manager and the other gentleman. I was so ashamed; I never let it known what I thought happened to those two ventilators.

Despite what might have taken place, I never gave up. I also never told anyone what I thought took place when I sent those ventilators. The thirty or more computers that I collected, I never sent them. I was afraid of what might have taken place. Before going on any further I must tell you what happen. The shipments were to arrive in two months times, but no trace of my shipment was ever found. I contacted the shipments yard in Durbin South Africa, but no answers. I called doctor Hlengwa, he too could not find out what happened to that shipment. Now looking back, I failed to go back to the shipment yard in Brooklyn, NY to get an explanation. I was so motivated to travel to South Africa; going back to the ship yard escaped my mind. Deep down inside me I felt that they were involved in a sham. I believed that my shipment was probably stolen and sold on the black market. You can imagine how I felt. I was in a deep daze. All of my thought about helping out the community and the hospital in Hlabisa South Africa had a good outlook, but circumstances like this made me doubtful about who to trust. Along with the computers I had collected, I also started to collect children clothes. Children were the most vulnerable in this worldwide epidemic. Here in America, children wore their clothes for a short period of time, then out grew them; leaving back clothes in good conditions. I went in my car to wherever I could go to meet such needs.

At work I started to ask for used children clothing. In doing so, I have traveled all over the city to pick up clothing. Doing this made me feel good. I was not doing this to impress anyone, just answering the call to help humanity. We are such a bless nation; things that I have collected were like just out the store. Had I not collected them, they probably could have been thrown out in the garbage.

I was at work when I saw the computer hardware being changed. I investigated to find out what they were doing with the old computers. I found out that they were going to be thrown out. Well, not all of them if I can do something about it. I went and spoke with the supervisor for that department. After speaking with him, he arranged for me to pick up as much of the computers as I needed. Now take a look at this, what could be more exciting than sending over to Africa, computers that could be of help to children in school.

To get started, I rented a van and went to the hospital I worked one early morning to pick up the computers. It was me by myself; I did not seek to get any help. I cannot forget that day. I had to park the van outside the hospital. Then go to the security for a clearance pass in order to bring the van onto the premises. After doing this, I then went to drive the van under this dark basement. This is where exchange of material going in and out of the hospital took place. Why do I remember this so clearly? This was where a van came to pick up a body for the funeral home. I was not afraid; what I was doing was to help improve lives and to make a difference in the lives of children.

Picking up these computers was some task. I was here before and I looked at all the ones that might be good. I did not want to pick up any of those that might not be in a good functioning condition. I wished I had gotten someone to help me; however, I managed to get about thirty computers or more. I drove the van home and called my dad to help me unload them. A few weeks had gone by when I called my brother who is a computer engineer. I told him that I had collected a few computers from work to send over to Africa. We both arrange a time for him to come and see them. To my surprise, he told me that something was missing for these computers to work properly. He told me that these computers need a mainframe to send them information. By themselves they were useless. Unlike my home pc that is connected to a printer and can be connected to the internet, these computers I had collected could not do that on their own. Now I was disappointed and felt used. I thought that each of these computers could function on its own. This would have been good for different class rooms to have their individual computers. After getting over my disappointment, I investigated the true functions behind these computers. The fact was that in a business setting like a hospital, computers received and sends out information from a central location.

As I traveled on this caravan of love, doors started to open spontaneously. I happen to get a phone call from Ed and Sunny. They wanted to talk to me about my plan traveling to South Africa. We all met one evening after work at a location in Manhattan, not far from Lexington Ave and 70th street at a restaurant. We all had a small meal while we talked. I shared how long I have been working as a nurse, about my family, motivation that got me involved with the HIV/AIDS crisis. One of the things that I shared with them, which is still true until this day, is the fact that no one that I know including myself is infected with HIV/AIDS. I know of no one with this crippling disease. The closest I have came to knowing someone is by taking care of them as a patient. Usually in cases like this, knowing someone usually helped to motivate an outsider to take action to help a circumstance. My motivation was unexplainable. I have been lifted up on a path that has taken a whole of me. I explained to Ed and Sunny why I would not put down this mantel very easily. I went as far as to say that I would like to visit this little town in South Africa. I told them that I did not have the funds to make this trip. Previously I had looked up the price for a trip to South Africa and it was very pricy. At the end of the dinner Ed and Sunny told me that they would sponsor my trip to South Africa.

Now I must tell you that I was lost for words. In all honesty, we do not know each other. This was the second time we were meeting. The only credit I can give myself was that I spoke very honestly and I allowed myself to be seen for who I am. Ed and Sunny are international business people. In my mind I thought that you do not impress such people in two visits. Just like you right now, who have been reading this story, you too have gathered an interest that I cannot explain. There is something about this story that is different from many others you have read. You may or may not be able to explain what it is, however you too have been caught. Just like I have said in the beginning, this is a caravan that I am taking you on. You cannot get off until you have fulfilled your purpose in life. Now this is one of my purposes. Have you discovered what is yours?

In this one moment, I had a loss of words. That moment in time, I began to thank God for his wonderful work and making a way out of no way. When I first started on this project, I never could have thought things would work out this way for me. I had all hope and expectation, but I never thought it would have taken this path. I have called quite a few travel agencies, went online to find a plane ticket to travel to South Africa. The cheapest I remembered hearing was 2300.00. I do make a fair salary, but reaching this goal would probably take me another year. I thank Ed and Sunny for helping me make this dream come through.

A few months ago before I met Ed and Sunny, I thought going to the South African Council at the United Nation would have been a big help. When I got there, I asked to speak with the supervisor. She was not available at the time. However, someone else spoke with me. I told her about the news paper article I read and the devastation HIV/AIDS was having in South Africa. I told the representative at the time that after reading this article, I felt obligated to do something. I am here to see if the council could sponsor a round trip to South Africa. At the moment, she told me that she would relay this information to her supervisor. I gave her my telephone number and email address. About two days after I received an email from Miss morge. She complimented me on taking on such a task. However, she could not send me on such a mission.

Ironically on the same day that I visited the South African Council, our Secretary of State Mr. Powell was speaking at the United Nation against Iraq and the potential problem it poses with weapons of mass destruction or WMD. The entire world was captivated by him and what he had to say. We are all living in a perilous time; we fight and kill each other instead of talking things out. The secretary's talk that day was to motivate and get the world ready for war. Some would say that only a few months before this day, we were innocently attacked; whoever did it need to be punished. We cannot allow innocent people to be killed without retaliating. They have weapons of mass destruction and they need to be stopped. I believe in eliminating all weapons, weather they are nuclear, biological, political or HIV/AIDS. The less time we spend creating weapons of mass destructions, the more time we have to deal with devastating diseases.

I too developed a slogan of my own about the war I am fighting. I called it WMDD. HIV/AIDS is a weapon of mass destruction and despair. Though the world called radiological and biological weapons WMD, there lies a weapon that all of us being fighting for many years and still many may not even knew about it. I tell you what WMDD mean to me: the tragedy of reading about children suffering because mothers and fathers were dead from this disease. This sometimes leads to children growing up without parents, young children taking care of their younger siblings; communities unable to supply or support those suffering from the illness of HIV/AIDS and hospital services unattainable because the fee cannot be attained by the needy. The shame and despair one suffers if it is known that they are infected. Children left in the hospital to grow up because mothers have this virus, and is unable to take care of herself and baby. Some children are unable to attend school because no one is there to support them emotionally or financially. The national government does not recognize this disease as existing. This is what I called WMDD. The war against HIV/AIDS still continues. You are now traveling on the caravan with me; you are the ears and eyes of those afflicted by this disease.

There is a WMDD. I hope you play close attention to what I am saying. We are here to awaken the world's attention to this devastation. One of the simplest things you can do is to buy a book or make a donation to the HIV/AIDS fund wherever you are. The word richest powers may not have been paying attention but we are here to draw their attention to this crisis. There comes a time when courage cannot be given, but is earned through the hard work one endures. You will join with me through this journey. We do not live alone; we all live and share common necessities to make life more enjoyable. We cannot stay by the corners of our comfort zones and allows this tragedy to go on unmatched. We need world leaders to sound the bells of raging thunders so all the world will become aware of this disease. We are fighting against a disease that compromises us from a vulnerable vantage point. As human beings we exist by sharing and giving love; we are not fully functional until these needs are met. We too need to strategize a way to fight back against this disease. Modern medicine has enabled us to live longer and healthier. In this case, the very young to the very old are vulnerable to this disease. I give world leaders something to come together and fight against; WMDD.

The way we fight against this disease is by using all the means that we know. We are having a late start to a disease that has affected and infected millions across this globe. I am willing to sit on an international panel to discuss some of the ways we can fight this disease. We need to communicate to the entire world about this disease. There will be some difficulties to over come, such as knowing at what age this level of communication should start. However, ever since this disease has started, a new generation has come along. We cannot wait any longer. All nations should come with a unified voice dealing with this disease. From communication we can consider going into developing different way of dealing with the immediate impact this disease is having. We need to consider the financial, medical, psychological, lack of education, and social impact this disease is having. We have fought many wars but this is a silent war that has no code of ethics or compassion. Let me remind you that we are all vulnerable in more ways than being infected. I worried about the world my two sons Jadon and Jonathan will live in; if not for yourself, aren't you concern how we are leaving this world for the future generations? We cannot settled that we cannot do anything more to improve the future. Despite all the troubles we are going through now, we have to take a stand and make ourselves accountable for actions we have taken. We are still on the caravan together.

The last time I met with Sunny and Ed was at a restaurant. Now I am invited over to their apartment. I was greeted by Sunny at the door. They have a beautiful apartment. At first I was shown around the apart; this made me feel very comfortable. I can tell that Sunny loves to read, she has lots of books. I feel less nervous as the evening went on. A nice meal was made for me. After eating, we got down to talking about going to South Africa. Ed had been to Africa many times. He shared with me things that he experienced. One of the things that he mentioned was the need for crutches. Many innocent people had succumbed to land mines and had loss a foot or partially paralyzed. This conversation made us connected more. Here I was in the home of someone I did not fully know, yet they have opened up their hearts to me so much. This is something amazing. Now talking to Sunny and Ed, I cannot afford to be unfocused.

Leaving their home that night, I saw where I needed a focus group. There were some things asked of me I did not know. Such as how would I know things sent over was going to the right people. The New York Times reported Rachel had given me doctor Hlengwa as a respectable person I could trust. However, I do not know doctor Hlengwa myself to attain to his honesty. How would I make sure that they receive the things sent to them? There were other questions asked of me; however, these lines of questions made me became more focus.

I started to call around to get some feed backs from friends and family, even coworkers. The most interesting and interested person I spoke with was Lisa Nelson. We worked on the same unit together, now she had moved on to another hospital. After telling her about the events that has gotten me this far with South Africa, she too developed an interest in visiting the country. This made me felt good. Lisa and I began to developed strategies on how to make going to South Africa a success. We talked about bringing gifts such as t shirts, candies, and toys. This was for the children, those in the communities and those in the hospital. We talked about finding out equipments the hospital may need. We decided not to focus on the big things, but more so things that will be beneficial to the children. I still cannot forget this meeting. It was like we were studying for an exam. This happened at a small Spanish restaurant, Hillside Ave and 179 Street, Jamaica NY. We got a lot accomplished. The next time I met with Ed and Sunny I brought Lisa with me.

Lisa has always been an enthusiastic person that makes a room lights up. On that evening she did. On this evening Ed and Sunny had brought few of their friends over to her home. She had someone that worked in banking, business and others. The room was delightful with people coming together helping us. We had dinner, talked about life's events, AIDS, and my trip to South Africa. We had an educational evening. Everyone had something to contribute to the evening dinner. I was told that not all American appliances worked in South Africa because of the voltage. They can work with a converter. We had conversation about different charities that would support causes around the world. I was asked questions by the group and they supported me. I got lots of encouragement. At the end of the evening, everyone was anxious about what I would bring back from South Africa to talk about.

A few days later Lisa and I spoke. She decided to go on the trip with me. I do not know what pushed her to make that decision, but I was happy. I had told her that Ed and Sunny were going to pay for my ticket. She wanted to know if I could ask Ed and Sunny if they could pay for her ticket. I told her I would ask, however, I did not feel comfortable asking them to pay for her ticket. At the time, I was caught in the middle. I needed the company but I did not think it was okay for me to asked Ed and Sunny to pay for her ticket. I do not know how I developed the nerve to ask but I did and was told no. After I got the answer I told Lisa that it was not going to be possible for Ed and Sunny to pay for her ticket, but if she still want to go, I would pay half and she pay the other half of her ticket. We both agreed that we would go that way paying for her ticket. At the end I was happy the way it worked out. This is what we should have done instead of asking Ed and Sunny to pay for another ticket. Paying for Lisa's ticket gave and showed a level of commitment we had to making this trip.

I brought the money for Lisa's over to Ed and Sunny's work place. When I got there, Ed and Sunny were not available at the time so I gave the money to their son to give to them. I was relieved that everything was happening. I felt like a little child waiting to open a present. I do not know what this trip will be about, but I hope the best will come from it. Yes, already a lot has come from this journey. The caravan of love once again has lifted my faith. When you believe that something can happen and it is about to happen, it takes you to a different world. Traveling to Africa for the first time had a profound impression on me. I would be the first out of my family to travel to Africa. Traveling to Africa is not strange, but in a sense it is because I am a black man returning as a stranger. This should not be the same for my children and their children. I will make it a place where we visit as often as can be.

Here I am about to visit a land ravage by so many horrors by the hands of human cruelties over the years. While at the same time, here we are hundreds of years later with another plague killing innocent people in this same land. Taking a look at history, it seems the more we move forward, the more we go back to the hands of relentless sufferings. Hundreds of years ago the hands of the superior race killed and conquered innocent Africans. Today we are going through a similar rage, where biological virus is killing so many innocent people. Little has changed throughout the years to calm the hearts of African. Although I was not born in Africa, I am a descendant of that land, and also have carried many of the old scars that linger on. I am very happy that I am going to Africa, but I cannot ignore and allowed the shameful pass to go unnoticed. I am happy I am on the caravan of love. This caravan will be there for us when we feel alone or being ignored by those around. We all need an added boost at times to strengthen the inner man. As we travel through this lonesome path, we cannot ignore those who have traveled down the same path. I can imagine men, women and children tied up on lonely boats threading through rough seas, having lonely days and nights to be their guide to far away land they knew nothing about. Well I am about to make a journey that will forever impacted my life. Though it is a calmer sea and I am traveling by air, this journey cannot be ignored or cut short; I am on a battle with full speed ahead.

The flight was a night flight leaving JKF international airport in New York. We left around eight thirty that night to arrive the following day. This flight would take twenty hours; with one stop in North Africa. At the time, South Africa was eight hours ahead of us; this made it interesting. Going we would loss eight hours but coming back we would gain it back. We traveled in a very large plane. The looks of people traveling that night were much diversified. There were blacks, causations and many other nationalities. This was my first time traveling to Africa; I did not know who to expect seeing on this flight. A part of me was scared; not outwardly. But I had some concerns about the outcome of this trip.

This was not like traveling back to Jamaica where I expected family and friends to greet me at the airport; most interestingly looking forward to that first homemade meal. In this case I was secluded to my own expectation. I listen to the music provided on this flight. Entertainment was up to your own discression; you can choose the movie or the music you wish to listen to. I believed I watched all the movies and listen to the music of Usher over and over. Along with the entertainment, the food was very good including snacks. Because I worked in the medical field, I often take frequent breaks and walk to the bathroom. I do this to prevent built up of blood clots. Whenever I got up to walk, I saw lots of friendly faces which calmed my heart; I must be going somewhere where people are nice. After about ten hours the plane landed and there were exchange of passengers and a new flying crew came on. I must tell you that I was a little restless. The most I have flown before was three and a half hours and I was in Jamaica by then. I remembered closing my eyes after we took off the second time. I was out of following the correct time. I told myself that I had made the first ten hours, I can do it all over for the second.

I must tell you, unlike traveling to the Caribbean on an airplane, traveling to South Africa were a smooth flight. When I started this trip it was night in New York, and again I am about to land in South Africa it is night again. I started to feel the smooth breaking of clouds although I could not see any. The announcement came over that we were approaching Johannesburg airport. After awhile I started to see spots of lights below. At this moment my heart was filled with joy. I am about to put my feel on the soil of the continent of Africa. I must tell you that this was big for me. Throughout my life time I had heard so much about Africa; even to the point where I always wished I could find out which part in Africa my ancestors came from. I am back traveling on the caravan of love. We had a smooth landing. Preparing to come to South Africa, I did all the research possible. I looked up the currency, time zones, and took precautionary medications. Looking at the people about to leave the plane I knew I had overlooked something in my preparation. I noticed the people were putting on coats. I thought only warm and hot weather in South Africa. When I stepped outside, I had a chilly welcoming; the weather was about thirty five degree. This chilly response made questioned myself; why I did not know this. I can tell you why, when you think you know something, often times you ignored everything else.

Despite this misunderstanding, I had no doubt. I knew this trip was meant to be. Well I have landed, and that is a fair question to asked, however I know the answer. We are here together on a journey that will change your life and your perceptions about people. We spend the night in a hotel and got up early the next morning to catch a connecting flight to Richard Bay, South Africa. Where we spent the night was not far from the airport. A shuttle bus picked us up and brought us to that terminal. We checked onto a small planed that carried ten passengers the most. On board they served a small breakfast; I ate and made myself comfortable. My eyes could not resist looking down from above at the trees below. Like a Roman's soldier they stood strong and green with a beautiful swing from side to side. Looking at them, I knew if they had eyes, ears or lips they could tell stories that would amaze many. I believed these trees were hundreds of years old. We finally landed at Richard Bays airport; a very small airport. We got our entire luggage; it was probably eight a.m. After getting off the plane I tried to contact doctor Hlengwa. After a few tries, a Good Samaritan was passing by and helped. I was able to speak with him. He told me he would send someone to come and pick us up. He told me the color and the model of the car the person would be driving; not very long after we saw the car. We went over and introduce ourselves and started on our way to meet doctor Hlengwa.

Chapter 3

DAWN OF A NEW BEGINNING.

BEFORE MEETING DOCTOR HLENGWA for the first time, the natural fear of the unknown over took me. I hoped within myself that everything would go well. I had already made the commitment to travel across the globe, but here I was in a daze. I have never done something like this before. I am a quiet person, and I hoped my inner strength will elevate me to a level that even I myself would never expect. It is not that I am not sure of what I am involved in, but at this point I am fearful, concern that traveling all this way will not be a failure. Being here in South Africa is a success by itself; but something needs to be gained from being here. I do not want to look back in my older age and can only talked that I visited South Africa when she was going through her difficult times dealing with one of the world's most deadly epidemic. I want this trip to be remembered as one where innocent minds come together, great things can get done. The news paper article below helped me to realized that what I was engaged in was helpful and beneficiary not only to myself but to others also. When I read the article below, I saw doctor Hlengwa as a vulnerable young man, almost so as the patients he cared for and the communities living in fear. The news paper article helped me to understand and to pursue higher achievements. Join me once more as we see and feel what one man is going through as he tries desperately to bring hope and restoration to a people living in fear and turmoil.

"AIDS Obstacles Overwhelm a Small South African Town

By: Rachel L. Swarns
The New York Times, March 29, 2001

Here is a summary of this article. This article shared with us the desperate need for help by people living in one community in South Africa. Things we would take for granted, people living here were desperate for. One doctor servicing his community was like an angel sent from above. His name doctor Smangaliso Hlengwa. To the communities he served, there were none like him.

He stood against those who were denying the root cause of the deadly cause of HIV/AIDS. While medications were limited to those who need it, he found a way to obtain these medications for his patients; because he knew something was going on many were not embracing.

Because of his stand along with others, the drug companies started to cut the prices on these antiretroviral medications. Where ever he could get samples of these medications, he would do his best to give to his patients. From his practice, he observed changes in patients who had the opportunity to take these medications. Although he was doing this, majority of his patients were not able to afford these medications.

"South Africa has 4.7 million people infected with H.I.V., more than any other country, and officials here are confronting a crisis of unprecedented scale, an epidemic far larger than that of its neighbors. Botswana has 50,000 H.I.V.-infected people who need treatment; South Africa has 600,000 and that number is only expected to rise.

"I tell them, 'Hang in there. Keep on trying,' " Dr. Hlengwa said of his patients, who must often choose between buying food, paying school fees and buying medicine. "I say, 'There's good news, the drug prices are going to be reduced. One day, it will be better."''

While encouragement is welcome, many longed for an answer, acknowledgement of the truth, and promise of the elected officials to find an answer. A handful of people like doctor Hlengwa alone cannot continue to fight this crisis by themselves.

According to this article, doctor Hlengwa has hope for a brighter future. This battle will not continue to be neglected. Doctor always encouraged his patients to take care of themselves the best they know how.

Reading this article gave me courage that the person I am going to meet will be someone I can work with. It tells me that this person has respect and faith in the improvement of human dignity. People working in the medical community have hope for a brighter tomorrow and faith that their hard work will make a difference n someone's life.

I have only spoken on the phone with doctor Hlengwa a number of times, but I had never asked him how old he was; I was anxious to meet him. The driver slowly pulled up to a gate where I saw a young man walked out briskly. Within myself I could not believe he was doctor Hlengwa but with excitement in his legs he walked up to us and introduced himself, after this encounter I had no doubt that he was doctor Hlengwa. He came over to the car and greeted us with hugs. Yes it was doctor Hlengwa; he was young man. He was taller than me, fair complexion, he had a little belly, and he dressed very neatly. From where we met, he brought us over to the Africa center, a private lodging. I do not remember everything we did on that first day, but I remembered we started to plan our daily activities right away.

I was impressed with doctor Hlengwa's approach to our visit from the start. He is a doctor, but there was something more impressive about him. To me, I got a feeling as if the world was going to end tomorrow. But in reality looking back, this was a young man who was witnessing something he himself as a doctor had no control over. He was overwhelm and showed it in a passive way as he encounters us. In all honesty, I come to understand that he has seen a lot of the sufferings the people not only in his community, but in his country and around the world were going through an health crisis, help needed yesterday. This sense of hopelessness had turned this young man not into someone who is easily given up, but into a fighter for his people. With our presence, I can see the presence of hope on his face and the thankfulness that something good can happen when you don't give up. This young man was in a sense of amazement looking at us. Talking to him on the telephone, I could never tell the sense of urgency he had for help for his people. Going over the different locations he wanted us to visit, showed the level of involvement and dedication he has for a better tomorrow. Because the Hlabisa Hospital was one of the sites written in the news paper article, he wanted to take us there including community centers, other hospitals and homes in the community. Doctor Hlengwa had left private practice, and was now working with the mayor of the town of Metubatuba; the mayor was someone we would meet.

Doctor Hlengwa was excited that we had come to visit South Africa through these troubling times. He was fascinated to learn how I got involved with HIV/AIDS. I told him that before I read the news paper article in 2001, I was a protectionist against this disease and had no outlets to get involved with this crisis. When I used the word protectionist, I mean I do not get involved in risky behaviors socially or sexually. I am a prime target because I work in the health field taking care of patients with known and unknown medical issues. Like I have said before, I knew of no one with this disease. I am not here in South Africa because I had a love one succumbed to this disease and I am here out of respect for that person; I am here because of the love in my heart and to let those suffering from this disease know that people out there love and care for them.

He told us that from a young boy he had grown up in the ghetto, but worked very hard to become a doctor. It was not easy but he believed in himself.

This HIV/AIDS crisis is worse than apartheid. With apartheid, we were separated but together. Now it seems as if we are all vulnerable and the leaders are not with one unified voice. The president of South

Africa does not believe the HIV/AIDS concept; he blamed it on something else. Behind that belief, many innocents' people are taken advantage of setting them to believe in the spirit world. From the short time we had spent together, I had gotten to know a lot about doctor Hlengwa. We both believe in the scientific approach to combating this disease as well as the humanitarian outreach that is needed to help the vulnerable ones. This was a good beginning because the last thing I wanted to know was that my trip to South Africa was unsuccessful because of unrealistic approach being taken.

We were at the Africa Center lodge where we would spend our stay. Breakfast and dinner was provided along with our lodging. All of this expense was covered by doctor Hlengwa. The lodging was clean and comfortable. At the front gate was twenty four hours security guard. The building was comfortable heated. In the living room was an entertainment set where you can watch television or use the computer. The dining area was separate with a long table and wooded chairs. You do not have to make your bed when you get up in the mornings; someone comes and made it for you. I felt comfortable with everything so far. The telephone system was different, but nothing beat calling our families back in America. We used calling cards which worked just like ones in America. I thank God for making this trip possible and the kindness of my friends Ed and Sunny. As you can tell, we are on the caravan. Nothing or no one can stop us now. The road maybe rough, but with love we will all make it.

The following morning we woke up and had a good breakfast to eat. The young ladies in the kitchen were excited to know that we were from America. They knew a lot about America. They tried to find out more from us about America. That was exciting; we tried to do the same to them also finding out about Africa. Doctor Hlengwa was waiting on us to finish breakfast to get started on our way. The first place we visited was the mayor's office. The mayor was very happy to see young people coming across the globe to learn more about the crisis of the HIV/AIDS was having in South Africa. After leaving the mayor's office, we went to the bank to exchange some money. One US dollar was equivalence to 1.6 South African Rand. Looking at the people around, they looked like anyone in America. People were walking going to and from their appointed locations. Within myself I looked at the peaceful nature of the people; I am thankful for all the hard work that made it possible for me to travel to South Africa as a black man. Here I am on a different path, riding on the caravan to show love to those suffering from HIV/AIDS epidemic. I am thankful for this opportunity and considered myself worthy to be here.

We traveled to a town where they were having a cultural function. It was a big function and a learning experience for me. Here in this town, we were in the presence of royalty. I did not know that there were royal families living in South Africa with honors just like other royal families in other part of the world. We were told not to look at the king directly and in his presence we should acknowledged his presence with a bow. I sneaked a peek at him, he was a black man. I got to understand that his reign was from hundreds of years through his family. The function was festive with music playing and people talking and dancing all over the place. I was at a royal function, but in my mind, this function was for me returning back to Africa. The food was a lot; and I hate. The food was delicious.

I felt good at this function, but something was at the back of my mind puzzling me. I could not understand how these people were so happy in the midst of this HIV/AIDS crisis. I questioned how they were able to make themselves so happy, even though I am happy that they were. You see I have traveled so far expecting to see despair, yet in my presence it was not so. Now I am not disappointed. I am relief to see in the midst of one of the world's greatest crisis, people can find ways to make themselves happy. I have shared with you about the caravan of love. The caravan of love was here with them. I did not have to open my caravan of love, because they already had it to share with each other. No matter where you are, you can look deep within yourself and find a small pot of happiness, it is the caravan of love. When you find it, don't hide it, but share it. When you share your caravan of love with another person who has the same package, people around you cannot understand what is going on. I was beside myself when I saw so much happiness. I just joined in and make myself part of the crowd. You and I know how the HIV virus is spread. In this part of the world, there have been so many misinformations given about the spread of the HIV virus. It is often shared that the spirit world is the cause of this disease. With that information, I would not be happy or be found in a public gathering enjoying myself. I took from this gathering of people a sense of resilience of not allowing anything to make them sad. As a first time visitor to this part of the world, I needed to see that.

It gave me a stronger drive to fight for these people. Someone may say that in the presence of the king, everyone has to be happy, but the joy I saw and felt was genuine. In there world happiness meant everything to them. With the large percentage of people suffering from HIV/AIDS, I believe they are aware of the crisis around them. However if you did not know this, then you would not be aware. Looking out the car window as I was traveling back from the function it made me think about the people in these communities. They have gone through so much with government abuse and neglect; maybe what they are going through right now reminds them of the past. Suffering will come, but it cannot stay, it has to go away. With great political leader like Mr. Nelson Mandela still alive, there is always the thought that this is not the end.

This day has come to an end, but it is just the beginning of a life experience that waits. The following day we went to Hlabisa Hospital. This was the hospital I read about in the news paper. Here I am, so close to seeing this hospital; I could not wait to enter inside. The drive to the hospital was very long. We traveled through some open forest before we arrived to the hospital. We were told that different wild animals could be seen in this forest, even tigers and lions. We arrived at the hospital after about two hours of driving from the lodging. Doctor Hlengwa knew the staffs at the hospital very well; he had worked there in the past. He took us to meet the director of the hospital. He greeted and welcomed us. I could not wait to see this hospital. Before I share with you about this hospital, here is the news paper article I read that put us on this journey I will never forget.

This is the new paper article in the New York Times written by Rachel Swarns, November 26, 2001 that inspired me and sent me on this journey; I have come to call, The Caravan of Love. This day was like many other days, I got up, went to work. A sense of hope enthuse me knowing that I was there to help and inspire the sick. A deep obligation always guided me to do my best. I take great pride in helping the sick to regain their health without abandoning their aspiration to regain good health. This involves restoring one's faith in overcoming set backs without letting the sick feels threaten or disappointed. Helping the patients restore that profound commitment to them regaining their will to work hard is something I enjoy doing. I do not take total credit for helping someone restore their good health under the medical spectrum, but I do know that my presence makes a big difference. Standing up for human dignity, while someone is compromise medically, is what I do every day for the sick. As medical professionals, we do our best at life's challenges every moment of every day. Here is a summary of the newspaper article I read November 26, 2001.

At the Hlabisa Hospital in South Africa, the medical staffs cannot escape from the endless horrors of witnessing the daily deaths of young men and women as a result of the HIV/AIDS epidemic. The medical staff cried endlessly for help but there was none. There seems to be no escape from this endless dying. The dedicated medical staff, they too wondered about their own safety. The government and the medical community were having conflicting reports about what was going on.

Despite the chaos that was going on, people were dying as if they were leaves dropping from tree branches. There were no out right confirmation of what was going on that could put the nation at ease. The daily horrors were more frightening, even to the medical communities. The sick out numbered the capacity to provide a bed. Despite these frightening occurrences, the staff at the Hlabisa Hospital did the best they could. Although frighten themselves, they brought cheers, songs of upliftment and encouragements to themselves as well as to the patients.

Since the spreading of the HIV virus, the hospital has an increase in the younger population of the community coming in for similar occurrences. Occurrences that identifies as symptoms associated with the HIV virus. Despite the back and forth that was going on about the cause of this illness, no one had true answer to stopping this crisis. Dilemma such as this needed a strong voice of comfort, not one creating more chaos. The entire communities were frighten, because there were so much suspicions of what was causing this disease, while no one knew for sure.

The medical communities knew what was going on, but they were limited in what they could have done. At the height of this epidemic, the president of South Africa was out spoken against the medical evidence that was available. False report was given to the nation by the government.

Regardless of the failure to inform the nation, there were voices speaking out against the epidemic South Africa was going through. Apparently, not everyone listened to the false claims that were supported. The call for answers grew louder and louder. Yes, painful admissions had to be made. The world we live is5 not isolated. South Africa was always looked upon by the outside countries. It was difficult to ignore the call for help, from a nation so desperately needed it. No one expected South Africa to under go another set back so recently after overcoming one not long ago.

Failure to identify HIV/AIDS as the cause of increase in deaths, led to many failures. The antiretroviral medicines were reluctant to be obtained. This would prove them wrong; no one in power ever wants to be proven wrong. Therefore many innocent people suffered and died because of lack of medical treatments. Believe me when I tell you that the HIV/AIDS is a WMDD.

The front line was at the medical facilities, doctors and nurses were limited in finding resources to fight against this disease. They were lost for worlds to comfort the families of the dead from this disease. I can imagine the stress that was placed on grief councilors, comforting these families. Despite all of this, the medical communities need more staffs to help run the hospitals smoothly.

Because of failure to admit the true cause of this disease, there lack of testing sights available to test people. Some patients ended up in the hospital when their bodies had become wasted; at this point the disease had taken a toll on them. At this point, you cannot escape the end result. They will die. Over seas the pharmaceutical industries are providing medications that are helping people to live healthier even though they remain HIV positive.

Help is available, someone need to take a stand. It will be expensive to medicate so many people; South Africa had one of the highest HIV/AIDS rates in the world. Many will call to God for help, but in all honesty, he already delivered the answer.

This problems or crisis got the entire nation frazzled. Parents are dying leaving there children with no one to take care of them. Infants born to a mother died while giving birth are left in the hospital to be cared for.

I was confided to myself after reading this article imagining the suffering these people were going through. Some changes are painfully obvious: the soaring number of admissions and deaths, the shortages of staff and beds, the general erosion of care due to shortage of man power and lack of general supplies making nurses and doctors struggle to conduct routine checks and tests. Reading this section of this news paper article stocked to my mind. The professional along with the people of this community are feeling the pain and suffering of this disease. There seems to be no escape from this plague.

While reading this news paper article you have a sense of the medical staff being overwhelm; overwhelm with constant death of young people the future of tomorrow. In this extraordinary emergency, there are little answers to the cause of this problem or a way out. Where help is possible, there are bureaucracy hold ups that seems to have no end or flexibility. The demise of innocence and increase in fear seems to paralyze this community. No realistic outlook can be seen coming anytime soon in this outcry for deliverance against this disease. Patients are identified by numbers instead of by their names which shows that sense of their identity and self-worth being taken away. There are more patients than beds available for a comfortable rest until seen by a medical staff. The shortage of medical staff brings about a sense of emptiness that even in the dying stage of a love one, they are receiving adequate care. Dying at home among love one seems to be a better way to this endless and tiring journey.

On the other hand, we do not know if lack of staffing is brought about by fatal demise of medical staff by this same disease. People preached that they have a cure, only to find out that the endless dying of young lives continues without any changes. Grief counselors themselves need assistance whatever way possible: antidepressants or migraine medications. The morgue is always full. Although some are sick with opportunistic infections such as pneumonia, they refused to take an HIV test; refusing to prove what might be an inevitable realism. This is my summary of this article. It is not easy to understand and even until this day I cannot say I do. I do not understand why some people suffer so much. Getting infected with the HIV virus is like been in war. The effects of this disease sure feel as if these people are in a war zone been attacked by those who suppose to rescue them. Believe me when I tell you this will not be the end; I will do what I can to bring comfort to this community. This I believe from the bottom of my heart. I ask for your help on his journey.

All medical facilities have a name, a face, and reputations to be respected and to transcend their works as leading institutions in helping the sick and the communities around. This was not the case when I visited the Hlabisa Hospital. The hospital has a name but her face was covered with poverty, suffering, neglect, shame, exhaustion, and stress. These were some of the emotional signs seen on the face of the medical staff that could not be hidden as you talked with staff members at the hospital. Imagine people would come to work to help take care of the sick, yet they themselves had to live with all these despairs; it was all around them. A hospital is somewhere people go to recover from illness and look forward to some restoration of good health especially when the sick person is young. All around people had to deal with the despairs of life. When they traveled out into their communities they continue to see and hear the same thing they see every day in the hospital; it's like there is no escape. The only escape is not to be a victim of this illness that paralyzes so many innocent people from the very young to the old. Despite all these people are going through they go to work because something in them will not allow the weight of this crisis to dictate their future; I believe going to work for them helped them pulled together. In a quiet way, the caravan of love gives inspiration despite all the chaos these people have to go through. When you have someone or something to inspire you to meet the task ahead, it brings about hope for tomorrow.

We visited the pediatric ward first where we saw children from infancy to about age nine. There were children there running around, some playing with each other and other laying in their cribs. There were some children there confined to their cribs; unable to move because they have become paralyzed. By not having that supportive environmental, social and emotional stimulus to move around, children became deprived of that needed developmental stimulus to forge ahead. This was painful to fully comprehend; as a father of two children, I felt these children were neglected. If a child was born paralyzed from birth, then I could understand why their movements were limited. However, as healthy children grew older, children move around. With limited resources, these children became victims. They became trapped in that web of developmental neglect and fall prey to the circumstances around them. These children have no parents and so they are left in the hospital for a better life. Ironically, the hospital has so much limitation due to financial restraints and lack of families coming into the hospital to help these children, some of them became victims. These children's mothers died from the HIV/AIDS crisis or mothers left their children behind because they were unable to take care of them. There was this one little boy who followed us wherever we went in the hospital. He had his little face painted with different colors. We had to stop and shared some candies we brought along. Like a little innocent kid, he laughed and enjoyed his candy. The tour guide informed us that the chances of a child getting out of the hospital are rear. Meals are provided for these children with daily change of clothes and medical treatments are provided.

To be abandoned from birth is a terrible thing. I used the word abandoned, because in a small sense, these children are abandoned, even though they are taken care of by the medical staff at the hospital. The long lasting effects on these children will be immeasurable and in some cases fatal. Look at the debilitating effects it has on some of them; words alone cannot explain these effects; and some of these children will never be able to completely explain themselves. We have that responsibility to raise the hands of those who cannot or those who are silent because of their sickness. We have the responsibility to make someone feel what love is. This is a treasure we cannot put a value upon; we have to be thankful that we know better and continue to do better.

The next unit we went to was the respiratory cluster. Here patients are treated for TB and other respiratory diseases. HIV/AIDS brings about a compromise to the immune system that makes people vulnerable to opportunists infections normally their body would be able to defend. In the TB unit, there were no separations from one bed to the next. Both male and female were put together in the same open space. Now this is very bad. There need to be separate quarters for each patient. Not having this patrician imposes these infections to spread to the next person and to those walking around.

The nurses and doctors taking care of these patients are also at high risks becoming sick because they have to go from one patient to the next without proper protections. In cases like this the inner human spirit ignores all signs of danger and pursues whatever it required to beat the odds of getting sick. This is call courage; the health care workers worked because they do not know when they or a family member will become victims of this relentless disease. In the shadow of the unit, the color of one's skin did not matter. All shade of health care workers black or white, worked together for the good of humanity. When you looked at the population of the sick these young people are suffering from opportunistic infections. Looking at the sick suffering, makes you do whatever you can to help them recover.

This is the respiratory cluster unit; however something runs inside of me when I see all these sufferings. When you look at someone having difficulty breathing, for a brief second you get caught up in their ailment. Just imagine suffering to breathe air something that you do not have to pay for. It does take your breath away just to know that someone right next to you is having difficulty to breathe while you are not. AIDS does not just takes one's life, but it make one suffer by different mode of sickness, then takes credit for it. I can imagine that these young folks did not plan to spend this time of their life like this. Just the look alone on their faces tells the suffering they are going through. For some it maybe the regret of not knowing why they are going through this torture; while for others it may be a generational curse. Whatever the case maybe, people should not be placed in a position where it seems hopeless; this is what you see when you walk through these wards. So I left this unit feeling sorrowful and hopeful knowing that despite all the set backs faced by these people, hope is ahead.

Next to the respiratory unit was the morgue. The morgue presented itself to us even if we had tried to escape it. You see, the morgue did not have enough space to accommodate all the bodies, so the mortician had to rotate the bodies in the refrigerator to the outside, to keep the bodies fresh. Outside in an open space of the morgue, were bodies covered up waiting to be refrigerated. When I saw this, it brought an ache to my heart. I was not afraid of dead bodies, as a nurse I cared for the sick and respect the dead. Observing what I was looking at was a total disrespect to the dead; however, what other option was available? The answer was none. There was no need to build a bigger capacity morgue when you only have eight deaths per week. Now we are in a crisis, where we all have to make compromises. People were dying from natural causes as well as from the AIDS epidemic.

When asked about the age group of the dead, seventy five percent were young people in their twenties to thirties. The other astonishing report was that there were more young women than young men dying. It is sad to see the young generation of any community die; this ongoing crisis puts a dark light on the future. Another sad thing about the morgue was the fact that they did not have proper containers to put these bodies in. The containers the bodies were placed in were like man made crafts/containers, wheelbarrow used to move the bodies. This was an insult to the dead but this was only a path to escape the crimson life here on earth. To the mortician this must be an endless parade of the dead. I did not ask him how he feels, but this cannot be enjoyable. One must take pride in the work he or she does, but in this case, it is troubling to see the bodies of young people parading for their final resting place. The mortician seems to be a man in his forties. It's difficult to tell the true age of a black person but I did not ask his age, instead I gusted.

I did not want to spend a lot of time around the morgue; it made me very sad to see so many young people bodies lying in a state of never returning. As a young person and a black man at the same time,

I am caught up in the thinking process wondering what if I was apart of this community. I know I would have been scared and frighten to have a personal relationship with other people, even having an intimate relationship as any normal young man would like to engage in, but all this would be frightening not knowing who to trust. This was how I felt. Now think about what I was going through. This only puts me in the same positions most of these young people must have been going through. What do we do as human beings when we are frighten and scared? Well, we seek the comfort of another human being. Maybe this is what happened to most of them, I will never be able to tell. There is one thing I know and that is for us to put an end to this plague that captures ones mind, body, soul and spirit. I look at myself and I feel so afraid and helpless. If this is happening to me an outsider, I can just imagine what the people in these communities are going through. I tell you, this is a war we all need to fight together. We cannot say let them go through their struggles. We need to help each other fight against this weapon of mass destruction and despair.

Across from the morgue was a little hut approximately seven feet by ten feet; inside here was the HIV/AIDS counseling office. Counseling was provided here along with testing for the HIV virus. The counselor were very informative and knowledgably about the HIV/AIDS crisis. They provided medical support, mental encouragement, emotional support and outreach in the community for the people. For a small place they have a big responsibility to the community. What I notice is that these employees worked well with people who came in for counseling; it like everyone felt vulnerable to what is going on. This little outreach center is a bridge to the community. This is where someone can go when they run out of ideas of where to turn. Families or friends cannot give the peace of mind this clinic can give when you are tested free from this virus.

Chapter 4

A CALL TO ACTION

ONE OF THE SETBACKS to this community is the financial burden and the medically underserved population. Not everyone has a job and many do not have medical insurance to pay for these screenings. This should be looked at carefully. If there could be out reach support to help the under privileged be tested, then many would know if they are HIV positive or not. I have been looking at the community, but the federal government need to play a big role in getting the population tested and encourage treatments. One in three women in these high risk communities is infected. Women tend to find out that they are HIV positive when they become pregnant and went for their routing maternity checkups; at this time it is found out. This is very sad, because at this point, three persons are at risk: mother, father and baby.

The South African government needs to take a proactive approach in talking to the people and providing medical treatments. There are other African nations that are facing similar medical setbacks, but because of the approach they have taken, the HIV rates are not as high as in South Africa. I believe the HIV/Counseling center should be much bigger. Once people are educated they will not end up in the morgue few feet away. In the counseling center, there should be doctors, nurses, councilors, social workers, pharmacists to give the people a full understanding of what is going on. I believe that people are fearful and not knowing where to go for information. They are only hearing a little at a time and by the time they hear the full story they are very sick.

I believe this approach would be accepted because people would not feel as if they are in a doctor's office. They would be more relaxed and able to absorb more information about the disease process and what needs to be done. Nurses are always needed to act as buffers. Things the doctors said to patients that they did not fully understood, nurses can explain more openly to the patient. In most cases, nurses will be from the same neighborhoods the patients are from; this would make the patient feel more comfortable in talking to them. This allows for more identification of resolving issues that patients need to get solved. Councilors are needed to help family with children get other family members to help; if a will is needed or someone to adopt a child, these issues can get worked out. Social workers can help families get access to medical insurance or food supplies in the home. The pharmacists can help alleviate any fear a person might have about taking certain medication. Maybe after taking certain medication, one might feel sleepy or nauseous, this should be explained. This is only an observation I am making to help people in the community reduce their fear of the health care system around them. I believe an up front approach is better than waiting for the sick to be buried.

I am not one to impose myself on a sovereign government; however, changes need to be made to the approach of taking care of people during this crisis. We cannot think that giving medication alone can solve this problem; an all rounded approach is needed to help solve this problem. We cannot forget the need of volunteers. Money is difficult to come by, but there are older people in the communities that are willing and capable of doing many things to assist those in need of medical care or food shopping. In many of these communities, we have melt down of the social order. In many cases both or at least one parents is dead. In other cases, the man, the head of the house hold has to work far away and does not come home until the end of the work week. We can regain these imbalances by having the community help one another.

This was the hospital I read about that brought me to South Africa. Seeing it in person was not like what I read. Words on paper cannot fully explain the enormous need that is needed in this hospital and in the communities around. I am asking for you to get on your caravan and get started; please join in, in this fight. Get started doing something for an AIDS/HIV outreach center close by in your community. I can tell you that the people in these communities are exhausted with the every day care of life and maintaining the basic fundamental of living. Living in a home with no mom or dad is frightening; when dad is gone mommy is always needed.

This is what I call WMDD (weapons of mass destruction and despair). This disease comes to destroy all fiber of resistance; it starts at the core of society, the family. We are called to fight for the survival of humanity. How do we do this? We do this through joining the caravan of love. These circumstances can no longer hold us in bondage. We are able to escape from this paralyzing episode that can not go on forever. In our fighting no one will get left behind. We will only left behind these horrors of circumstances that belittle us. For the first time I am proud to let you know that I am one of the captains of this ship. You too can be a force that diseases or circumstances of life finds difficult to recon with. Together when we all join forces and calls out to mother earth, we can force the despairs of life to disappear. We can do this; we are doing this right now. Just look thirty or forty years ahead and imagine what you see? This living hell cannot be allowed to continue.

Most bacteria and viruses existed on earth before us as human beings were present, yet we forge ahead and coexisted. There must be a way where we can go back to our peaceful way of existence together or by ourselves. This disease has found many ways to kill us; we must do the same to kill it. It must be a thing of the past; we too must find a way to destroy this virus. I am optimistic, but I do have some doubts. As human beings we find so many different ways to kill each other, instead of spending the time to love one another and fight for the common good of us all. If we change our focuses and look five years ahead, I believe we can make a big difference in the fight against HIV/AIDS.

You may say that I do not have what it takes to join this caravan. Too much is going on in your life right now. Well, you have done well so far reading this book! You have incidentally joined the caravan without realizing. Here are a few tips: accept yourself for who you are, give self credit, develop positive self values, accept your strength and your weakness, do not be afraid to make mistakes, turn setbacks into victory, join groups that promote positive self-esteem, demand respects from others, seek fulfilling love relationships. These are some of the positive attributes we offer on the caravan of love. If you do not have them we won't reject you joining; many of us are still working on one or two of these characters. As your captain this is my stimulus package I am offering. It won't cost you or left future generation tied up in a deficit. Ignoring it will leave us all to an uncertain future. Once again I asked you to join the caravan of love, make this world heaven on earth.

We visited a boy's school which hosted approximately one hundred and twenty boys. The ages of the boys ranges from ages eight to fifteen. Here the boys gather to gather to received us. They were happy to have visitor; however when they were told that we were from the United States, more joy appeared on their faces. It was doctor Hlengwa's idea for us to go and visit this site. We brought candies from the US which we took with us on that visit. It was amazing to see how fast the boys took those candies away from us. Later that evening when we went back to the hotel, doctor Hlengwa asked us about the day. He wanted to know if we had noticed anything different about our trip that day. He later explained to us that they boys tried to take as much candies as they could, because for some of them, that would be a meal. This made me sad. To know that a candy could serve as a meal for a child is unbelievable. I reflected on how much others take for granted, while a child in other parts of the world goes to bed with nothing to eat.

The next site we visited ran by a lady whose name I cannot remember. She visit homes of children who lost their parents or who has very sick parents and the children are left to be head of house hold. She has a group of seven women and two men. The females are about in their late twenties to sixties. The two men looked like they are in there mid thirties; they are the drivers and security for the ladies. This group has developed one of the most enriching programs to help children who are in need. They organized adults in the community to work with the children. During the afternoon after school, members of a community would work with children to plant crops of vegetables, and other greeneries. The adults would reap the crops and bring them to the market place during the day. Whatever money they make from selling, they would give to the children to help them purchase food and other items in the home.

When I look at this system, I can only think of ancient societies developing a system of commerce with other people around. It is a very good system. It helped provide financial support for these children. It gives these children an opportunity to talk to an adult. Despite the emotional and psychological pain they are carrying not having their parents, they have adults that are there with them even for a short period of time. We went and looked at one of these farms. I was impressed with what I saw. They organized different groups to do different tasks. There is a group to carry water to water the plants, another group to reap and prepare for tomorrow's production. Others were there to water the roots of the plants. Everyone comes out a winner from this organization. This too helps the children to develop organizational skills, communication skill and respect for each other. They learn different group dynamics that makes the work easier. They share information by communicating with each other. Each group talks with the other. I do not know if they do rotations of different jobs; this too would have been helpful to give a sense of what the other person has to do. They are the next generation in a world where you need another person. From what I see, they are doing well in an environment where everyone needs each other to exist.

After a long day we went home and returned the following day. The next site we went to was the home of two teenage sister and their three siblings; two of the young children were boys. They had no outside support other than this group of adults that goes around and checked on children who lost their parents. When we arrived, one of the big sisters was on her way out to the social office to see if they could get some financial help. We asked how successful she may be. What we heard was frightening. The South African government does not help a family such as this one as easily, but would do so much faster if one of the bigger sisters was pregnant. This was outrageous to someone with logical thinking. The person who is now pregnant is more likely to have contracted the HIV virus than one who is not. I think it make more sense to help these young children who are left to fend for themselves, than to allow them to be taken advantage of putting them at risk to get other sexually transmitted diseases. This gives rise to the question, who in the government is making and enforcing these policies. This is no way of providing aid to the needy, only putting these innocent children more at risk than helping them.

While at the home of these children, I notice the shy look on the face of one of the younger kid. He was about nine years old. He covered his head and part of his face with a hooded sweater. At first I thought he was just a shy kid, but when I took a closer look at the little boy, his face was filled with sores. Despite all the sickness going on in these communities, something else was going on with him. This little boy was suffering from malnutrition and without the necessary nutrients; his little body was breaking down. You cannot look at the outside of these children and ignored the entire person. This was the family we gave some t-shirts we brought from New York. This little boy needed someone to love him and to make him feel good about himself. He needed the right nutritional intake to help him fight against these second hand infections. They also need a better place to live. Where they lived was a one room made of dirt, where all of them lived together. It is depressing because so much is left on the children to do when they need their parents to be there with them. More and more of this occurrence is happening where mother and father are dead and children are left to take care of each other. In the social network in South Africa, the black man has to travel very far to work. So far that wherever he works he has to work and find a place to live during the work week and return home on the weekend. During this time while he is away from his wife and children, some men sleep around with other women, sometimes exposes himself to STD's. He comes back home infected with the HIV virus and gets his wife infected. Now in one home a man can have more than one wife, with each of the woman having children for him. A man can come home and infected both or all of his wives leaving them all to die from this disease including himself; leaving all the children parentless. Children with both parents dead suffers lots of set backs from lack of a loving home, good social family development and having good nutrition.

Malnutrition was one crippling finding that I discovered on visiting the families at one of the homes. This can be an innocent set back that does not present itself until keen observations are made and taken for closer observation. According to an Uptodate article on February 3, 2010, entitled "Malnutrition in developing countries: Clinical assessment" by author Buford Nicholis, MD. Section editors William Klish, MD, Kathleen J Motil, MD, PhD. Deputy editor Alison G Hoppin, MD. "Severe malnutrition is primarily a problem in developing countries. Severely malnourished children typically are brought to medical attention when a health crisis, such as an infection, precipitates the transition between marasmus (a state of nutritional adaption) and in kwashiorkor which is adaption is no longer adequate. This characterized by marked muscle atrophy with normal or increased body fat. For MARASMUS symptoms you see: Diminished weight, emaciated and weak appearance, bradycardia, hypothermia, and hypothermia, thin dry skin, redundant skin folds caused by loss of subcutaneous fat, thin, sparse hair that is easily plucked."

Most of the time, children go unseen for malnutrition until a crisis appears. The reason for this is clear; these children are only given essential food to eat when it is possible, because of financial or other restrictions. A professional clinician can make keen observation on seeing a person for the first time. Certain physiological evidences are presence on observation without blood test which can further confirm malnutrition. The body tends to preserve the function of vital organs by shunning supplies from less essential ones. The larges organ of the body is the skin; most of the time it is one to get deprived first.

Some of the evidence you may see in a child are: dry skin, loss of hair on the head, chapped lips, decrease moisture to eyes and mouth, diarrhea, bleeding from the intestines, decrease urination and generalized body weakness. Children and older adults usually become sick easily. Immediate medical attention is needed. This may include hydration and given adequate nutrition.

Furthermore emerging from these communities are the guilt and sadness when children are left behind because of the death of one or both parents. This is a delicate transition young children has to go through when their parents died. They are left with the uncertainty of who will care for them. They are bombarded with emotions of vulnerability; they may not know who to depend on with activity of daily living that they never thought about while their parents were alive. Trust comes into play finding people they can trust and depend on without being taken advantage of especially if they are very small. During these tender developmental moments they need someone to help them go through different stages of sadness and helping them to move on. The death of a parent can leave an emotional deficit on a child that if not dealt with promptly and effectively can last well into their adulthood. They must be given the chance to grief and be nourished with love and understanding.

The truth must be told to them that their parents will never be seen again and things they used to do will not happen any more. Children should encourage not to think about the death of their parents, this is only adding punishment to their lives as they grow older. The child or children must be observed for unhealthy behaviors such as being withdrawn for a prolong period of sadness. Behavior such as these can lead to suicidal ideations which must be dealt with appropriately. It pays to pay close attentions to these children; it does not matter what age they are, to loose a parent is devastating enough. This is a delicate period when young children should be protected and sheltered with love.

The effect of the HIV/AIDS epidemic has a well rounded effect on those that are infected as well as innocent children who has to grow up without proper nutritional support and social development because of this disease. According to the American Dietetic Association, HIV/AIDS Nutrition Therapy, include the following guidelines. Good nutrition can significantly improve the quality of your life. It keeps your body working well and support your medications and other therapies. Good nutrition also helps with other concerns, such as high blood glucose and body shape changes.

You will want to write down how much food you ate and what you weigh. Ask yourself these questions and talk to your doctor and dietitian to help you improve your nutritional status:

- Have you gained or lost much weight during the last year? How much weight, and during what amount of time?
- Are you having any problems that make you want to eat less or make it harder to get the benefit o the food you do eat? For example, have you experienced diarrhea, nausea, vomiting, loss of appetite, taste changes, or other issues?
- Do any foods seem; to cause problems for you? Which ones? What kind of problem.
- Do you eat a few meals every day? Do you have any problem getting food to eat? Do you ever go hungry?
- Do you exercise regularly? What kind of activities? How often?
- Do you know what to eat and not eat with your medications?
- Do you take any nutritional or other supplements? Which ones? Why?
- Do you have any other medical conditions, such as diabetes, kidney disease, high cholesterol or triglycerides, or high blood glucose levels?
- Are there any changes in your body shape?

First, find out he level of calories that matches your goal of maintaining, losing or gaining weight. Then talk with a dietician to get assistance when it comes to developing your daily food plan schedule for someone diagnosed with HIV/AIDS. The focus of your plan will be on high-quality foods. It will include a variety of fruits and vegetables each day. Fruits and vegetables have lots of vitamins, minerals, fiber, and antioxidants to help maintain your health.

Special Eating Problems

- To gain weight after an unplanned weight loss, you will need to address the problem that cause it (such as infection, loss of appetite, vomiting and diarrhea) and then eat well to replace the nutrients you may have missed.
- You may gain weight in unusual places. This happen when your body gains fat and fluid without the usual gain in muscle.

If this happens, don't restrict your eating. Instead, ask your dietitian about which foods to eat and other ways to work on this problem.

- Ask your dietitian for nutrition tips for diarrhea, nausea, vomiting and loss of appetite.

Grain servings	1 slice bread ½ bagel of English muffin 1 small tortilla ½ hamburger bun ½ cup cooked rice, pasta, cereal, or potatoes 4-6 crackers 1 cup ready-to-eat cereal	Good source of Carbohydrates, calories, a B vitamins. Whole grain are also a Source of iron, Magnesium, selenium, Zinc.
Fruit servings	½ cup cooked or canned fruits, oranges, banana ½ cup fruit juice 1 cup raw leafy vegetables	Follow food safety Guidelines for raw Fruits. Good source of Vitamins and minerals, fiber, antioxidants.
Vegetables servings	1 cup raw or cooked vegetables 1 ½ cup vegetable juice 2 cups raw leafy vegetables	Follow food safety Guidelines for raw vegetables. Good source of vitamins And minerals, fiber, and antioxidants.

Milk and Dairy Products servings	8 oz (1 cup) milk or yogurt 1 ½ oz cheese 1 ½ cup frozen yogurt or ice cream	Use pasteurized products. Good source of protein, calcium, carbohydrates, B vitamins, and minerals
Meats and Protein Foods servings	1 oz cooked meat, chicken, or fish 1 cooked egg 1 oz nuts 1 Tbsp peanut butter ¼ cup tofu, dried beans, lentils, or peas 2 Tbsp hummus	Best source of protein, Good source of B vitamins and minerals 3 oz meat is about the size of a deck of cards.

You can use this Food Group Planner to determine how well you are doing each day and where you need to change your eating habits. For example, if you had a meal of a grilled cheese sandwich, milk, and carrots sticks, you have consumed 2 grain servings, 1 ½ to 2 dairy servings, and 1 vegetable serving. After you have recorded everything you ate for a day, looking to see where you need more from a food group and where you might cut back a bit. Good nutrition promotes a healthy life style. This include having enough rest, having enough sleep, exercising, eating right and making adequate follow up with your doctor.

The next site we went to ran by two men. They have an open invitation for children to come in for breakfast, lunch and dinner at their canteen. They cater to the children whose parents are very sick and not capable to make a meal for themselves or their children. They allowed the children to take food home for parents who are very sick. We spoke with the young men who run this kitchen. The government and the community provide some financial help for them to run the kitchen; however, they never had enough money to meet the need of the community. In a little room where children sat and eat, they make the environment as child friendly as possible. They use colorful paintings to make the place come alive for the children. The seats and tables are painted in bright friendly colors. When you sat down to eat something, you are taken away to another place. Looking around it helps you to forget about the outside, while making you at peace with yourself. For the children who can make it, this is helpful. Whether or not this was the intended purpose, it helps serve a purpose. A purpose no one can take from you, while you sat and have an enjoyable meal. If a child does not show up for a meal, they investigate what is the cause of that child absent for that meal. I can see on their faces that they are tired but not forsaken. When they spoke they have a commitment to the greater good than over some frustrations. They were happy to see us knowing that from so far away, someone cared. Someone care to come and take a look at what they do, not for themselves, but for others around them who are not strong enough to cry for help.

HIV/AIDS is a WMDD (weapon of mass of mass destruction and despair) phenomenon that needs the world community to join together as one to fight it. No one nation should be going through this. I believe the more people join together fighting this disease; the brighter the future will be for finding a cure. I approximate the ages of these two young men to be in their late twenties to early thirties. Yes what they are doing is important, but they could be living a more productive life in society. I know from their presentation, they do not get enough money to do what they do. They could have been top chefs, yet they chose to be helpers to the needy around them. I would love to see these young men again to tell them to their faces that I am proud of them.

This weapons of mass destructions and despair comes in so many different ways to take advantage of someone when you are vulnerable and susceptible. This crisis does not only kill, it puts the entire community to suffer. Young people are set back from fulfilling their dreams and aspiration in their young lives. The social pressure it leaves behind put those around in better positions at risk for developing stress. It is impossible to walk by a neighbor's house knowing that he or she is sick and doing nothing to help. Young children are left to fend for themselves at a time when they need to be children. You have a break down of social norms that will take generations before it can be considered normal. I have one questions in my mind, how can these children grow up to compete in this advance global economy? Who takes up the responsibility of getting them back on track? I tell you this, I believe help is on the way.

We have no choice; we have this responsibility to do something to make the world a better place for these children. It does not mean engaging in something you cannot manage, as we come together with our caravan of love, more will be identified that can be done. A box of rice, used children clothes or new ones, used children toys or furniture all will be helpful and encouraging to these communities. When all may look bleak, there is a bright light around us that can send hope and inspiration to the less fortunate. You may not be able to help the hospital, but you and a friend may be able to do something for a community outreach. We are traveling on this caravan of love that will not stop until we reach the less fortunate ones.

This canteen was the last official site that we went to assessing the need of the communities suffering from the HIV/AIDS crisis. With an open eye the suffering still goes on everywhere you go. It's a never ending plague that festers to the innocence of those that are most vulnerable. Living in this type of a community requires one to have an enduring spirit. As much as one obtains the drive to move forward, something else usually comes and shatters that expectation. When you are not physically nourished, it takes a toll on the entire human body. Looking from the outside might not give a full depth of the enormous desperation one has to go through from day to day. There seem to be no escape because each new day seems worse than the last. When you look around, everyone seems to be going through the same thing. What a tragedy it is to born in a world like this, seeing everyone suffering with no escape. This is no good for a child. All the days of your life, nothing seems to be going well. Those children who lost their parents, with no one to guide them along the way are even more troubling. Imagine for a moment if you had to grow up in an environment like that. Maybe you do not have to imagine something like that because you are going through something similar.

Remember a while back when I introduced you to the sun and moon. No matter where you travel, there is a guiding light that is watching over all of us. You might ask the question, what happen when there seems to be more night around than day light? You can look up at the moon. There might not be much light from the moon, but still the moon is sharing the reflection of the sun shining on the other side of the globe. We have to remember that bad things seem to always present themselves, but faith augments the presence of something good. No matter how low we might be, we have to develop that zeal to reach for something better. It's no accident why I started on this journey. It is no accident why you are here on this trip with me. The caravan of love is more powerful than you and I can imagine. It gives us access to part of our being that empowers us to rise above circumstances around us and to release an enduring source of power. Though you may be going through a dark day, there lies a ray of light shining through.

You are not traveling alone on this journey. We are all one body; we cannot afford to ignore a part. We are working together for the same cause; we all have a function and a role to play in this endeavor. These families are depending on us; no one can fulfill your role in this path. I encourage you now to take a stand. You are now traveling on the caravan of love. You have little time to second gust yourself. You can imagine what these families are going through from day to day. Remember when we started out and I shared with you the never faded lights that accompany us wherever we go. You may fell alone just about now because the whole world seems to be running away from you. They cannot hear the calls you are making, the loneliness you are feeling or the cries you are making. When you look up or around, there is no light. You are probably thinking that if the sun is not shining then the moon should shed some light. Well, here what you need to do right now. Take a deep breath and exhale; there is no light around you because the light you need to see is deep inside of you. You have to believe in yourself. You have to believe that you have enough power to generate a light so bright, the world will be running to you.

The world needs to have a place to hide itself. All the time it was looking for that light too, so the good of humanity will not escape us. When Mother Nature seems to be sleeping, wake yourself up knowing that within you, you have the power to make this world a better place. The world won't tell you of its short come; it will only wait to see if you discover them. Despite what you are going through, you should not surrender. You are a strong person that has a lot to give to this world. Don't believe you are a failure if death should arrive unexpectedly. You are a winner; you will be at a place where these suffering exist no more. It was painful going through, but now you are free. So now you know that death brings about freedom and redemption, so let's fight with all our energy during this gifted time of being alive. Unleash your inner strength by believing in yourself. You have being doing well so far traveling on the caravan. Put a little love to your daily tasks and rise above unwelcome circumstances.

Chapter 5

LOOKING FOR A BETTER TOMORROW

I HAVE JUST VISITED a small community where the older adults take children after school and have them plant vegetables to sell in the market place when the children are in school during the day. If we had a caravan of love in this part of the world, things could be much different. I believe these big farms owners could make some financial contribution to the poorer communities. They could assist with irrigation instead of people carrying water on their heads to irrigate these vegetables. Maybe they could send around a van to help transport the vegetables the children planted to the market place. They could help with fertilization. This would have the children spend more time in school. Maybe they could recruit children who are interesting in farming to have an internship in agriculture. Yet as you look and see what is going on; you can see that things are one sided. These ideas may seem to be fragile social safety nets that may not mature to be of help. Please remember ideas are dormant until one makes a loud cry pushing them ahead. These may not be the best solutions, but they are one means available to take a stern look at finding helpful ways to awaken people to move ahead. When people join together to obtain a common goal, things that seems impossible become part of the regular routine.

We have to try and get back to a place where things are more balance; where everyone is represented equally. Continuing this display of unfairness will lead to a future of inferiority and superiority complexes where one group is dependent on the other. We do not need this, we need each other to come together and work with each other. The beneficial end result for both sides should be dual positive effects where no one feels left out, but is more codependents on each other. This requires a level of mutual engagement on both sides whereby no one feels threaten. This will lead to a positive development of mutual understanding and both sides will take time out to learn from each other and about each other. How do we go about this?

We start by generating love and respect for each other. Doing this will lead to an immeasurable result of dual positive effects; resulting in both sides coming out as winners while relying on each other. How is this achieved? Both sides have to focus on each other and the end result of benefiting themselves. There need to be openness and respect for the other side. Rising awareness of positive acquisition of resources should not be ignored or belittled. Developing trust should be so strong that a third party mediator should not be needed. Each side should encourage the other in exploring future discoveries that will benefit them both. Take for example economic independence should be encouraged so that more blacks could help each other and become less dependent on the established economic delivery system. Remember I introduce you to the community that helps the children cultivate farms during the afternoon and take the produce to the market place and the adults sell the produce for the children during the day. They have been doing this for awhile now and I would think that they have developed a method to this system. Here we are looking at the advance development techniques the white community has developed for themselves. If the black and white communities could reach out to each other and help one another, it would be of great help to both sides. The whites could learn how the black people are able to plant without using pest asides and little fertilizer. This could be of great economic incentive for the white communities to practice. The black can benefit from having transportation provided by the white community to bring their produce to the market place, while on the other hand the white would gain financially as they rent these necessary items.

Economically, some black people in South Africa have been oppressed in their own communities. They have limited resources to make changes to their lives. You find acres of land being cultivated in their communities, but the land is not own by them. I believe given the opportunity to transform and to make working an economic upliftment within their own communities, this can be a primary survival tool for great empowerment. Given this, there should be no great difficulties in blacks helping each other to get out of depressed economic turmoil. I believe people in the black communities will feel more positive about themselves getting the incentive to move ahead. This can lead to economic independence and developing new ways to bring prosperity to their communities. These rising awareness is powerful in leading to socioeconomic development and community improvements. Engagement of people in daily activities around them invokes growth now and also with future generations. These young children are observing what is going on around them keenly. There comes a time when one has to move on. This will lead to a subtle shift that no one can explain. Southh Africans need to engage in positive dialogue that will be resourceful to each other. This is not impossible; by us engaging in a dialogue, we can over look and learns from our mistakes.

Traveling on the caravan of love makes the impossible probable. We can encourage an atmosphere of brotherly love that make people far away want to be like to be like us. It does not matter what nationality or religion you are we can work together for the common good of humanity. Time is waiting on no one. As you close and open your eyes, time continues to move on. The world is becoming a smaller place, despite no changes in square meters. You do not have to travel to South Africa to be of help. You can stay where you are and purchase items from there. This is sewing a seed of prosperity. The older females in South Africa use their hands to make many household items that can be purchase and put on our walls or food table. As we sat around our food table eating, purchasing an item can help someone else put food on the table and clothes on their backs. This can help send a little boy or girl to school to have a better education to help them prepare for the future. The eyes of man may be blinded, but the sun will continue to shine bright and the moon remains as a reminder that the sun never stop continue to shine.

Everyone in South Africa has a role to play in fighting this disease.

Doctor Hlengwa went back to his community to help; he did not stay away because he became a medical doctor. Help someone. South Africa is a beautiful place to visit. Help a person to obtain a job, help a person start a small business, help a community to open a heath center, help a community to send the children to school, help the world to see South Africa. No one can be blamed for the chaos this epidemic is causing. This is an opportunity for you to stand up together fighting this disease.

Chapter 6

JOURNEY BACK HOME

IN CONTINUING TO TRAVEL, we journeyed to meet doctor Hlengwa's family. It was very far from where we were staying; about two hours drive. Before we went, we purchased water some over the counter medications just in case we should encounter any sickness, and some non perishable food items. This travel exposed the beauty of the rural part of South Africa. There were trees that looked as old as two hundred years. The branches of these trees covered a wide span of space. The far look ahead over sees mountains and valleys. You cannot get enough of these magnificent sceneries. The further you travel, the more you get lost in these unfathomed beauties of nature's delights. The landscapes designed in many different shapes, gives way to its beauty in multi-demotions over lapping each other. The trees seem to wave their branches in a silent shout of greeting and welcoming us. The cool air eases their way across our faces, letting us know and feel the winter breeze of South Africa. I have never been to Africa before; so I ease back and enjoy the beauty and peace of this moment. The treacherous past these trees and the people of this region have gone through has not been forgotten; however, we can close our eyes and let the breeze blow on our faces taking us to a place of unspeakable joy and enjoyment of the beauty of this country. If trees could speak, they would take thousands of years to unfold what this beautiful land has gone through. So I welcome the silent wave of the tree branches that welcome a brother back home. I have been the silent one of the three of us; doctor Hlengwa exposed us to the history of the region as we travel.

On our journey we saw big cultivation of crops with irrigation systems watering the crops. Acres of sugar cane field and logs of wood cut down waiting to be taken to the saw mill. These were the works of white Africans. We were told that blacks had little to no parts in these regions, yet they live close by. Hearing this was not easy. We should all learn to share with each other. Here I am on a journey fighting to help people suffering, yet in their own land, they do not have a chance because they are being taken advantage of. It is astounding when you think of the controlling mechanism of this country. The blacks do not have adequate resources to cultivate the farms. They do not have the equipments to water the land. They do not have access to transportations to take their crops to the market. No trucks to take sugar cane to the factories.

We continue on our journey until we reach the home of the parents of doctor Hlengwa. Their home is located on top of a hill over looking the valley below and across wide land space. Some houses were made from brick but others were made from trees and barks of trees on the roof of the houses. The home of doctor Hlengwa's parents was made of wood casing, dirt floor and tree barks for roofing. This was not a surprise for me. Despite the make up of the houses, the people around were very happy. I could not speak or understood the language they spoke, but the smile on their faces and the way they looked at us, made me felt welcome. They did not have electricity in their homes, yet their love and happiness made their home well lit. We were introduced as foreigners from America, there to visit. They welcome us. During the night they use fire lamps with kerosene oil to see. The moon light is a big help in making the place look lit. From where I sat, you can see the light of other homes far and near making the surrounding looking like a bird nest of beautiful lights. Later during the night people gather together and start to sing and dance. They judge the rhythm of the dance making it a well participated competition among each other. You do not need to have a mechanical instrument to feel the rhythm of the night. Both old and young people participated in this family gathering. The night ended for me early because I was coming down with the cold and felt very sick. I went inside and wrapped up until the next morning. We went Friday afternoon and left midday Sunday. I learned a lot for the short time I spent there. The people appreciate the little things in life that most would take for granted. This was different from the busy life of New York. People were laid back and relaxed. There seems to be no care in the world that worth stressing over.

The calm of the night brings the entire family to gather in a circle invoking the start of singing and dancing. There are no age limits to this festival of family enjoyment. On the sides are lit battle torches; the moon light made the lights of the torches fade into a beautiful night. Each family member take turns in getting up and clapping and dancing. Each member tied to do a better performance than the other. Like passive judges we clap and cheer louder for those that do a better performance. Along with the dancing that is going on, tea and crackers are served to those around. This is an eloquent way of being greeted I thought to myself. It was refreshing to see the togetherness and the strong spirit of family. Looking at these people, you cannot deny that they enjoy life despite what is going on with the HIV/AIDS crisis around them.

I asked doctor Hlengwa about the HIV/AIDS epidemic in this part of the country. I was told that it does exist but not like in other parts. One of the contributing factors was that of socioeconomic issues. Some men have to travel very far to work with limited transportation, so they would stay away from home until the end of the week their work schedule ended. While they are away from their families, they engaged in sexual relationships with other women outside and bring back the virus to their families. Now, some of these men has two to three wives living in the same yard, in different houses. As you can imagine, coming back home infected, he spread this disease to all of his wives; leaving young children with out a mother, a father, financial support and most of all left to fend for each other. As I hear this it made me to think of a better socioeconomic structure that would made families stay together rather than driving them to destruction. I believe having a viable economic developed structure where people can work and come home can make a difference in the lives of these families. This cannot be done tomorrow, but a start can be made for improvements. This will bring about economic improvement as well as leading a constructive path in dealing with family unit and breaking the need for a man with three wives to go out and have an affair. A strong family structure is one of the key components for having a strong community. This will allow the children to grow up and be better than mom and dad.

Doctor Hlengwa is a prime example of changing the current way of thinking for improvement in the future. Not everyone would be able to leave where they live, but if improvement and development of economic structure can be made in these areas then that would be very good. What can be done in areas such as these? A developer might be able to develop camps, hotels, and restaurants where visitors can go. I would be one of the first to revisit this area. Jobs can be developed for someone to keep the place clean, clean around the ground of the camp, hotel staffing from front desk to laundry room. A restaurant always needs a cook and someone to clean the dishes. The world is a much smaller place today. All we need to expose this place is to advertise it and bring it to the Oprah show. Otherwise we can advertise over the internet. We can first start by inviting fellow African to visit these sites. We can offer free breakfast if you are awakening up by 8 a.m. This will turn out to be so relaxing. During the day people can be taken for tours; coming back they will be so tired, they will need to have a good night meal and a comfy bed to sleep on. We all need to get away from the busy life of the city and find a relaxing place to rejuvenate ourselves. Finding different ways to stimulate economic development in each community is good. This will help preserve the family structure while at the same time build a stronger future; this can be done. Family structure is preserved when men do not have to be away for a week before returning home from work.

One of the advantages of traveling on the caravan of love is to discover different ways to escape from potential disasters that come along on this journey through life. We are not immune from these potential disasters that creep up quietly. People find ways to climb Kilimanjaro one of the tallest mountains in the world. We cannot afford for fear to overwhelm us and keep us down. Think and act not for the moment, but for the children and families looking for stability to move on. A future of security and safety and the willingness to let go of the painful past can bring about a prosperous future; limitation faced in life can be overcome. We are not asking a lot, only for some passive economic stimulation; you will be fulfilled and enriched knowing that these communities gain their economic independence. You are needed on the caravan of love tour. We are all one body. We cannot afford to ignore one part over the other part; all the members of the body are vital. We are all working together for the same cause. We all have a function and a role to play in this endeavor. These families are depending on us; no one can fulfill our role in this pursuit. I encourage you to be a part of this journey. Pick something out and use it as an instrument of restoration.

Maybe you can think of some other ways to stimulating economic development in the rural areas of these provinces of South Africa. You can share these ideas with us. Some day in the future you can visit South Africa and see your ideas at work. You will be proud to be a pioneer on the caravan of love tour. Your journey on this tour is appreciated and welcome. You will not be disappointed with this movement of love and awareness of the suffering people with HIV/ AIDS are going through. Like I have said, the time was short but I enjoyed myself here. It has opened a bigger awareness of the need for education, health information and economic developments in many under privilege societies. I will never forget this part of the world. I plan to visit another time.

The return from doctor Hlengwa's family was quite refreshing and relaxing. We knew this was close to the end of our trip in South Africa. I have experienced more than I have expected. Despite all the sadness we have come across we have found time to laughed, cried, close off in corners by ourselves. On our way back we talked about the different experiences we had been through since we arrived in South Africa. I am a quiet person, but I was a little too quiet on our way back from this trip; while everyone was talking I was just there listening to them talking. Something got a hold of me and all I remembered asking doctor Hlengwa to pull over the car on the side of the road. I got out of the car and I started to danced. My hands were flashing, my waste winding and a big smile on my face. Flowing from my eyes was tears that I could not hold back. I was overcome with emotions of happiness, sadness and hope for a better tomorrow. The HIV/AIDS epidemic made me feel trapped as if I could not escape the daily horror of young people dying, poverty in the communities that made the people felt helpless or the lack of truth from their government. Here I was in Africa on a mission to help those in need. There were many before me that could have helped those in need but did nothing. Some tried, but got distracted. Others died fighting for equality. I felt free and happy traveling to Africa making an impact on improving the lives of the present and future generation here. This book is to share with the world the difficult things people are undergoing, yet so many are not aware. So I danced to relieve myself of unhealthy burdens, I danced because I am free, I danced to let everyone around me know that we are no longer in bondage or captivity, very soon we will all be able to dance. I danced so that those large trees could wave their braches suspended above the earth as a sign of restoration. I danced that one day those staff members and patients at the Hlabisa Hopsital will be dancing too.

The atmosphere in the car changed because of my dancing. We all laughed and made fun of each other. This was about seeing apart of me that was unexpected and unbelievable. Getting back into the car I felt refreshed; apart of me I could no longer hold on to. As I traveled along, I wished one day people all over the globe could have this sense of freedom and feeling safe. I do believe this will happen; it does not have to take another generation. I think the world has seen enough of the suffering from the HIV/AIDS epidemic. We reached back to our hotel safely and went for a good night sleep. The next day we went to Ghost Mountain where we met with the Mayor of the town of Matubatuba. This is not the first time we have met the mayor, but he wanted to talk with us before we return back to the United States. It was a far distance from Metubatuba to Ghost Mountain. We arrived safely the night and had dinner with the mayor. At dinner he informed us that he has a proposal for us at breakfast in the morning. We enjoyed dinner and went to bed. The hotel was a top class hotel; I planned to take my wife there in the future. The following morning we woke up and had breakfast with doctor Hlengwa, the mayor and his advisors.

We talked during breakfast but we got to the meat of the matter after breakfast. The mayor asked us to be ambassador of South Africa for the town of Metubatuba. He explained how proud he was of us reaching out to help others in need so far away. This Endeavour would include us sharing educational information, fund raising, involvement with economic development in the community and social education having to do with overcoming HIV/AIDS. We both listened and agreed to be part of this Endeavour.

I am burden by personal ambition as well as a great drive to write this book telling of the story many will find fun to hear. You have traveled through this war zone with me finding many WMDD's. We will not retaliate with weapons to cause destructions, but with love never seen before. I thank you for your commitment to this cause; traveling on the caravan of love. Like I have said to you from the beginning, there is no end to this book. For this book to end, then there would have been no beginning to it. Life exists on a circular sphere. If we are not careful and vigilant, we will make the same mistakes over and over and not realizing what we have done, instead blaming life's short comes on someone else. You have the responsibility to spread the word around about this journey of love for humanity. Don't feel as if you are alone; we are guided by our instinct of survival. When we are faint in spirit, heaven gates are always there to open up and guide us through if we allow it to happen. We are all surrounded by a force of energy that brings out the best in all of us.

Unfulfilled hope is a heavy burden to carry especially when young children are left to carry on by themselves without their parents. The thought of not having a mom or dad to guide a young child through life is painful. Young children need the nurturing care of a good parent. Most of the young children whose parents died, is left to fend for each other or for themselves, often time are left to make decisions that have grave consequences. The hope of having mom and dad being around is taken away. These children are left to make decisions about what to eat, wear, and their safety. This is all costly, and without mom and dad there to help, put this child at risk.

Chapter 7

AIDS/HIV VIRUS

WHAT ARE HIV AND AIDS? Human Immunodeficiency and Acquired Immune Deficiency Syndrome. HIV stands for human immunodeficiency virus. Once you are infected with this virus, you will probably be infected for life. AIDS stands for acquired immune deficiency syndrome. To get AIDS, you must be infected with HIV. The following are ways that HIV can be spread:

- Through contact with blood and certain body fluids (sperm, vaginal fluids and breast milk).
- Having sex (especially if not using a latex condom) with someone who has HIV.
- Injecting drugs with used equipment.
- An HIV infected mother may spread the virus to her baby before or during birth.
- HIV may be spread from a mother to her baby through breast feeding.

How is HIV not spread?

- Food, or sharing plates, cups, or silverware.
- Insect bites, such as mosquitoes.
- Sneezing or coughing.
- Swimming pools, or other public places.
- Toilet seats, clothes, or sheets.

• Touching the skin of a person who has HIV.

Don't believe that because HIV and AIDS treatments and medicines are improving, you no longer need to take precautions. These medicines and treatments are hard to remember, have side effects. They are expensive and needed for a long time, probably the rest of your life. Keep a written list of the medicines you take, the amounts, and when and why you take them. Bring the list of your medicines or the pill bottles when you see your caregivers. Learn why you take each medicine. Your medicines and other treatments may change often to better control your disease. This is often decided after caregivers see the results of your tests. Work with your caregiver to find the best combination of medicines to treat your condition. Do not take any medicines, over-the-counter-drugs, vitamins, herbs, or food supplements without first talking to your caregiver. Always take your medicine as directed by caregivers. Call your caregiver if you think your medicines are not helping or if you feel you are having side effects. Do not quit taking your medicines until you discuss it wit your caregiver.

Chapter 8

Needless Neglect

F OR MANY YEARS THE President of South Africa, denied the existence of the HIV/AIDS epidemic leading his nation into a devastating crisis. In a New York Times article dated March 7, 2000 by Rachel Swarns, "Mbeki Details Quest to Grasp South Africa's AIDS Disaster."

"Pretoria, South Africa, May 6—for months, President Thabo Mbeki says, he pored through medical journals, consulted with scientists and struggled to understand the epidemiology of the AIDS epidemic that is ravaging this country.

"I am reading all these complicated things, language I don't understand," Mr. Mbeki said today as he addressed an advisory panel of international AIDS researchers here. "I've got dictionaries all around me in case there are words that are difficult to understand. I phone the minister of health and ask her this word mean and she explains.""

Less calling and more listening and hands on needed in fighting this fight. President Mbeki had little to no knowledge of what was going on at the time. His refusal to open his eyes to what was going on in his country, led to more devastation itself that the spread of this epidemic. Head of the scientific community in South Africa blamed President Mbeki for failing to educate the public about the true scientific nature of this disease, instead of wasting time on unproven theories. This falsehood had led to misinformation to the general public. It was so bad where President Mbeki, seek false information from researchers who believed the true scientific data about this disease was caused by poverty and malnutrition were the true causes of this disease.

Despite President's Mbeki's failure to come to grasp with the impact of this deadly disease, the human concerns will not allow us to loss the focus on identifying this disease as a crisis of enormous proportion. The lives loss and destruction of family structures has taken many by surprise, leaving children to take care of children because mother and father have passed away by this dreadful disease. Believe when I say that our dedication to follow through will take us higher level and bring promises of hope to us all; ending this suffering. Despite shattered confidence to those around the world, those who are infected and those who are not, I bring comfort. The plight of this disease will be made know despite those who would like us to be silent. There are those who tend to profit from us being silent, but we will not. The time has come for us to suffer no more; we have suffered long enough without being comforted. The virtue of human dignity is crying for help; we can be sick but we should not have to suffer.

Former President of South Africa Mr. Mbeki failed to get a full grasp of the AIDS epidemic. In is failure to get a full grasp of the epidemic, he outreached to those with conflicting report on this disease. I find it difficult to understand why one person would resist and deny full medical access to millions of his people own people. Mr. Mbeki did not give researched and known knowledge a chance to prevailed and observed. Instead, when Mr. Mbeki could not find satisfying explanation for such differences, Mr. Mbeki began exploring the work of researchers who believe that poverty and malnutrition are more likely causes of the disease in Africa. It is so ironic that he looked at the effects of this disease as the cause. We have to be one step ahead of these reasoning. This is a leader that failed to reach out to his people. There is a lot that needs to be discovered about this virus, but ignoring proven scientific discoveries at the peril of your nation is ignorant. We won't regret not having a revolution against this government, because the damage is done. We have to save our energy for a bigger fight.

In a July 15, 2000 article written in the New York Times entitled "Focus on AIDS, Mandela Says", by Rachel Swarns "Closing the 13th International AIDS Conference today, Nelson Mandela urged scientists to move beyond their concerns about South Africa's president and to focus on combating the epidemic that is raging across the African continent."

This is what can be done. We need to get our communities, social groups, churches, political organizations, schools, work places and our governments involved. With the advent of computer and the use of the internet, this will be a big help. There is a need, a cry for help that many are not hearing. Medications are expensive, but if we can get a group of people to talk to the drug companies, then we can purchase a lot more for the under privilege. It makes no sense that a drug company can record billions of dollars in end of year profit, while a world of needy family is left to die because they cannot afford to take the medication they need. The vulnerable as well as the privileged are caught in the middle. Those that can afford to purchase their medications are charged extra and those who do not have the money are left to their own demise. All countries need to take a look at their societal priorities. You cannot afford to ignore your citizens' medical needs while you pursue other developments.

South Africa needs to rise to the occasion and come from behind the curtain of self-denial. The entire international communities know that HIV virus is the cause of AIDS. It is difficult for a country to progress forward in fighting this disease when the leader is ignoring the true cause of it. This does not give the people a clear focus on how to go about fighting this disease. The people of South Africa: blacks, Caucasian, Indians Europeans and other ethnicity groups. Not long ago you all join together and ended racial segregation. You are all needed again in this fight. The luxury of tomorrow depends on our hard work today, improving the quality of life for every citizen young and old. We have to come to unite on one cause, appreciating the dignity of human lives. We do not need leaders who might be, but leaders who will be more caring and efficient to making changes without being personally offended by making adjustment to the way they look at changes. I respect leaders who support the need to cross boundaries in order to support and maintain progress and long lasting achievements. However, despite President Mbeki misconception about HIV/AIDS, he was not alone, many scientist in the science community were lost and over taken by this disease when it was first discovered that such a disease existed.

Chapter 9

TWENTY YEARS OF THIS DISEASE

THE EDITORS OF THE above article give us a complete assessment of the HIV/AIDS epidemic over the past twenty years. Despite all the knowledge we have gained over the years, it seems as if we have not been able to have a full grasp on the seriousness of this disease. We need to develop a social approach that will help us to observe and take certain universal precaution to help stop the devastation and stop the spread of this disease. We are all responsible to limit the spread of this disease; the lease you can do is to talk about it and educate yourself. Continuing to live carefree sexually or socially ignores the human mission of living in a peaceful global community. We cannot leave everything up to the government alone or the pharmaceutical industries. We all have to take some responsibility in fighting this disease.

According to The New England Journal of Medicine, April 30, 2009. Paul E Sax M.D. and Lindsey R. Baden M.D. "When to Start Antiretroviral Therapy—Ready When You Are? "The optimal time to start antiretroviral therapy in asymptomatic patients has been one of the central controversies in the care of patients with the human immunodeficiency virus (HIV) since the introduction of the first antiretroviral agent, Zidovudine, more than two decades ago. Since then, periods of enthusiasm for aggressive early intervention have been followed by a more cautious more cautious approach.

For those who do not believe the devastation and the crisis the HIV virus is causing around the world, they need to pay close attention to the following editorials. On the website Uptodate, The global human immunodeficiency pandemic. Author Thomas C. Quinn, MD, Section editor John A. Bartlett, MD, Deputy Editor Barbara H. McGovern, MD. "While initially limited, infection with the human immunodeficiency virus (HIV) has literally exploded over the past two decades to become the worst epidemic of the twentieth century. With more than 35 million fatalities, the AIDS epidemic now ranks alongside the influenza pandemic of the early 1900s and the Bubonic plague of the fourteenth century in terms of fatalities. The impact of this disease on human suffering, cultures, demographics, economics, and even politics has been felt in nearly every society across the globe."

This epidemic continues to be a killer around the globe. No one can announce that they have not heard of this plague. From the young to the elderly, this disease has killed and continues to infect millions. Some parts of the world are more severely infected than others, given that; this disease needs to be stopped. Unfortunately, the epidemic continues to spread.

Children around the globe are greatly affected by this disease. Many have lost their parents to this disease; leave then susceptible to hunger, poverty, and lack of a good education. Enormous responsibilities are placed on financial stricken communities to provide ways to take care of new responsibilities. With such devastating global epidemic, I expect more from world leaders when it comes to fighting this disease. A lot has been done by the United Nation and other countries around the globe, however, its now thirty years since the onset of this crisis. We have seen the re4sults of moving slowly thirty years ago, why do we continue to move slowly?

There are some barriers that need to be abandoned; like those believed by President Mbeki. Common sense approaches could have done more than medical discoveries since the onset of this crisis. Education is the key to fighting this disease whether this generation or the next to come.

The discoveries of Antiviral medications have made significant improvement in reducing the life expectancy of someone diagnosed with HIV. Much more can be done to decrease the spread of this disease. The lowering of drug cost can be one way; another is to encouraging everyone to get tested for the HIV virus. Personally, asking for an HIV test result before engaging in sexual acts should not considered to be over burden. We have to become brave and aggressive when it comes to fighting this disease. It may not be popular but fear of the unknown is worse.

Chapter 10

BENEFITS VS RISKS

IT IS MIND BOGGLING when you discover the number of abortions taken place annually. I am not here to take a pro or con approach to abortion; however, if we as a society can take a more critical look at this approach, then we can make progress in reducing STD's including reduction in HIV acquisition. The fact that a woman is pregnant through the normal sexual encounters between a man and a woman automatically puts her at risk for acquiring STD's or the potential infection of the HIV virus. My take is that women who do have induced abortion also need to take into consideration that their lives are also at risk for acquiring HIV when engaging in unprotected sexual activities which does not discriminate. We need to reach a place in society where we need to understand that for every abortion pills or surgical methods exist the potential for both males and females contracting the HIV virus exist. Abortions may get rid of an unwanted pregnancy, but it does not take away the possibility of being or getting infected. As a societal need, we need to show and give respect to our sexual partners and ourselves where we present ourselves honestly to each other about our sexual histories and behaviors. There is no way a woman can know if a male is HIV positive if he does not let her know of his sexual history and both of them go and get tested for STD's. Now in the real world, no one has time for a long drama when it comes to sex. Therefore I recommend we get to know ourselves and our partners better, and have a meaningful relationship with one person. There need to be an awareness that AIDS can be forgotten but has not gone.

Every pregnancy is a reminder of the potential fatal acquisition of a STD affecting mother and the new born. Abortion will get rid of an unwanted pregnancy, but little can be done to get rid of an unwanted STD that you have to live with the rest of your life.

The AIDS epidemic is undermining the very social fabric of many cultures in developing countries. The demographics, economy, cultures, and political structures of many countries have been dramatically affected by the spread of HIV/AIDS. The challenges to controlling the epidemic throughout the world are enormous but must be overcome today and in the very near future. To meet these challenges, the development and worldwide distribution of inexpensive antiretroviral drugs must be supported; and the accelerated development and distribution of a safe and efficacious vaccine promoted. These is no doubt that the clinical science of HIV research has made and will continue to make a dramatic difference in this epidemic, but the initial optimism that followed the discovery of HIV, the development of diagnostic assays to help monitor the epidemic, the prophylaxis of opportunistic infections, the identification of effective antiretroviral drugs and the prevention of perinatal transmission has been tempered by the stark reality and magnitude of the global HIV pandemic. A concerted effort must be made from all international health agencies, philanthropic foundations, and governments from the national down to the community level to implement immediate prevention programs based upon education behavioral modification, and treatment of those infected with HIV."

Abortion is not being debated, nor is it looked at as a cause of the spread of STD's, however, it underscore the need for more community interventions to help women pursue healthier sexual intercourse. The pharmaceutical industries need to develop a vaccine to fight against STD's. On the other hand, women is not looked at as the main perpetrator when it comes to the spread of HIV/AIDS. A matter of fact, women are caught in very vulnerable position. Women are tend to be taken advantage of in socioeconomic deprived communities, when they have to be the bread winners and are not able to.

Chapter 11

REDUCING BARRIER FOR HIV TREATMENTS.

In previous chapters, we tried to show the social dilemma as well as the need for governments to rise up and take a stand against the spread of HIV and other STD's. I cannot claim that there is one solution to this epidemic. It is well over twenty years now since the acknowledgement of this disease. I believe there is something we can do to decrease the spread of this disease. The world is waiting for an answer; at this point in time, it does not matter who finds it, as long as it is made known. If a cure is not available, maybe we can develop another strategy in reducing the spread of this disease.

In an editorial in the New York Times entitled "Hope in South Africa" August 20, 2009 stated. "For years South Africa was an international laughing stock for its tragically absurd approach to the deadly AIDS epidemic. Now, that national nightmare may be ending. The new government of President Jacob Zuma seems to have a clearer-eye view of the problem, its remedies and the need to improve the overall health care system than its predecessor did."

Years of denial and ignoring the existence of the HIV/AIDS crisis has taken a toll on South Africa. Many do not know how to go about fixing this problem. It has become more than a symbol of ignorance, but one of disgrace to this nation. The population needs to be informed about the true nature of this disease. Someone the people can look up to and trust because of all the hypocritical lies that had been fed to the nation over the years. The previous president, Thabo Mbeki, compiled a record that until today is still hard to make sense of. His belief and acceptance of false claims about the true cause of the HIV virus had placed South Africa back into the middle ages. Even when the truth was difficult to dismiss; he found ways to portray his thinking as the only way to his nation. I believe majority of South African citizens has come to accept the true cause of this disease today.

The new health minister, Dr. Aaron Motsoaledi, under the authority of the new president, President Zuma, has came out and accept responsibility for the prolonged failure of not acknowledging the lack of responsibility that had led South Africa in to a pit. He was encouraging at the same time, that as the nation work together, they will eventually rise about this disaster. Moving ahead wont be easy, but he believed South Africa will rise up once more.

According to Dr. Aaron Motsoaledi, he encouraged the leaders of the country to wake up and discard hypocritical ideas and to encourage the scientific communities to embrace sensible approaches went it come to fighting this disease. He made a loud cry to immediate attentions to be made to decreasing the spread of this virus from mother to child. In his view, this crisis has put South Africa under the spot light of shame and disappointments. He spoke of the risk factors that lead to the spread of this disease. This was important to announce to the nation, to let the people know that we are speaking with one voice when it comes to fighting this disease.

He acknowledged that the nation faced a big problem at the present time. There is not turning back; to continue ignoring this problem will only lead to annihilation. The problem is big but to has to be corrected. The government has to initiate improvement in the way the citizens access health care; at least once a year annual reporting to the health clinics. Let's start a fresh and bring about a brighter future. HIV/AIDS will never be forgotten; lets do all that can be done so it will never be ignored again.

The caravan of love tour offers the world an opportunity to think and act not for the moment but for the future for ourselves and our children. Though the focus of this book is on South Africa, the entire world is also vulnerable. We have to take responsibility in getting rid of the spread of this disease. It is so ironic that two of the most prominent nations on earth, the United States of America and South Africa, could find themselves in a nonchalant and procrastinating manner when it comes to developing effective and educational methods to fight against the HIV/AIDS epidemic. It is counterproductive for a leader of a country to inform his or her nation suffering from this deadly disease that a scientific explanation does not exist; or a nation failed to give medical treatments on a whole for those who are suffering from this virus. One nation has risen to the call and has taken a stand to fight against this global epidemic.

The New England Journal of Medicine, 354: 1977-1981, May 11, 2006 "Fighting HIV-Lessons from Brazil", by Susan Okie, M.D. "In the history of the response to the HIV pandemic, Brazil is best known for its pioneering decision in 1996 to offer free combination antiretroviral therapy to all citizens with AIDS. The government-funded treatment program, which some critics predicted would lead to rampant drug resistance, has been hailed internationally as a milestone in the fight against AIDS. The program has improved the health and extended the survival of tens of thousands of Brazilians, has saved the country an estimated $2.2 billion in hospital costs between 1996 and 2004, and has inspired similar efforts elsewhere-including the President's Emergency Plan for AIDS Relief (PEPFAR), whereby the United States provides AIDS drugs to African and Caribbean countries, and the World Health Organization's 3 by 5 initiative, which sought to provide HIV treatment to an additional 3 million people by the end of 2005."

No doubt the outside world has learned something from Brazil, who has taken aggressive steps in preventative action against the HIV virus. While other government officials failed to acknowledge the true cause of the HIV virus, Brazil did not. Give credit where credit is due. Preventative measures were developed and initiated. This included development of treatment programs and testing sites for the disease. Implementations such as these decreased the spread of the virus, improved the relationship between the government and the people; who included testing for the virus, many people are receiving government-sponsored antiretroviral treatment.

Condom use has also increased in the general population. Another issue was prostitution; in Brazil prostitution is not illegal. o more than $500 million by 2007.

When people say, "Tell us how to do it,' we cannot tell them.'" According to Google, the following statistic is made available showing the global epidemic.

Globally the HIV/AIDS epidemic has infected someone. From Asia, Africa, Europe, North America, South America and Australia, all across the globe the HIV/AIDS epidemic has spread. Some regions of the world have a larger percentage of infections than other. Even so, we are all vulnerable. Millions of people in each continent are infected with this and many have died also. Given all we know about this disease, a cure need to be discovered soon. Until such time, all precautionary steps needs to be taken. This disease is a weapon with no mercy to the innocence or vulnerable. We have to take a stand; this includes pressuring our government to take bold steps in reducing the spread of this disease.

Chapter 12

ELEMINATE RAPING & EMPOWERED THE YOUTHS

IN AN ARTICLE IN the New York Times dated January 29, 2002 by Rachel Swarns entitled "Child Rape Increasing at Alarming Rate in South Africa", gives credibility to the fact that people are turning to traditional reasoning and medicine instead of scientific approach to help combat this deadly disease. "Sinazo is 8 years old and doctors say she is so damaged inside that she will never have children. Her mother prompts her gently, and the words come rushing out. "He stripped my dress and my underwear," Sinazo says. "That man, he stripped himself. Then he raped me." Beside the spread of the HIV virus, this is one fight I am personally committed to help fighting; the raping of young girls for medicinal purposes.

Sinazo's story is not the only one, across South Africa; young girls are brutally raped by strangers as well as family members. This mentality has to stop; and it starts with the learders o this country speaking out. Speak up about the cause of the HIV/AIDS epidemic. Speak out against raping of innocent children; and bring justice to those who did swiftly and severely. Encourage community groups and parents to join together with one voice condemning such acts. Statistics may show increases in such acts, however, consolidations of voices can bring change and peace to innocent families.

President Thabo Mbeki, in his New Year's speech to the nation, confessed to the nation of the alarming increase of rape against children and the frustration the public has against non ending evil. He made it clear that this was a battle everyone needs to help fight. You can help in this fight by reporting cases to the authorities; take an innocent victim to the doctor. Do not be afraid to report a friend or a family member who are involved in such despicable acts. Everyone is trying to figure out what is triggering such insane behaviors.

According to police and medical reports, South Africa has one of the highest one of the highest per capita rates of rape and sexual assault. Such disturbing report made innocent citizens afraid and foreigners frighten to be in this part of the world. Looking ahead, something has to get done; and the answer is not when, but right now. The children are our future; destroying their future from such a young age serves no purpose.

It is strongly believed that someone who is HIV positive can get rid of the virus in their body by having sex with a virgin. Whether or not this is a reason for the increase in raping of young girls, it has to stoop. This is a civilized nation, raping of young girls has to stoop.

The civic communities of South Africa are showing increase interests in ridding the country of such bad statistics. Police officers are responding to calls of rapes with more arrests. The court systems and civil services are providing more assistance to rape victims. There are light at the end of the tunnels, but it should not have taken this long for something to have been done.

To little Sinazo, you will grow up one day to look back at these dark days you had to go through. You may become a lawyer to protect the innocence from the hands of the unjust. You may become a medical professional; ho help the sick to overcome their sickness. You may become a chef; let everyone enjoy a delicious meal whenever you cook a meal for them. You may even become the first female president of South Africa. Whatever you become, let love guide your life wherever you go.

All hope seems to be fading away from parents with their young children. They need to find a safe place to raise their children where they can grow up safely. As children grow up, they need their independence to go out and explore the world without having to be afraid. I pledge to the parents and families of South Africa, justice will come on the caravan of love although healing will come much later. In the face of impossibilities, we will overcome all odds and move to higher heights.

Everyone can see the direction and the turmoil the country is going through due to the AIDS epidemic. We need strong leaders who are not afraid to stand up for what is right. Those of you who have been following the plight of South African suffering from this deadly disease, have seen how those given the responsibility to protect, have neglected the innocents. From time to time it seems as if the people of South Africa are given spoons to empty the ocean. It seems this way because as they overcome one hurdle another one rises up and sometime it is more problematic than the previous. Something can be done and should have been done a long time ago to help the people of South Africa combat AIDS crisis. Just take a look at Botswana a neighboring country that has a higher rate of HIV infections. The government of this country has accepted the right sequence of action by providing medical attention for those suffering from this crisis.

Despite the despair the people are going through, Sinazo and her mom still have faith for a better and brighter future. The daughter believing in becoming a doctor and the mom believes she will have a better place for she and her children to live. No one wants their children to live in an environment where they are raped and laughed at. No sympathy for the victim or over the evil they have to go through.

The government of South Africa needs to speak out against these outrageous behaviors. This government should not want to be responsible for carrying on a legacy of abuse and neglect in their country. It is time for young and old to embrace the future with open arms. It is now time to regain your integrity and not to return to behaviors of the past. Raping innocent children is no different from what disadvantage were taken place under the apartheid system of government. I tell you that you need the young to stand strong to help carry the older generation. When you disgrace and shatter the hope of the younger generations' future, what hope remains? People in the communities need to join together in fighting against antisocial behaviors and also speak out against these criminal acts. Growing up I pledge to visit South Africa during my lifetime; this was during the apartheid rule. Now I had the opportunity to, I am disappointed to hear that black people are so cruel to each other. When I see a young child, I forget about the negative behaviors we as adults are capable of committing. I look on their innocence and would do whatever I can to shield them from the cruel world some of us allowed to protrude our lives and make the world a painful place to live.

The aim of this book is to help find different means to adapt to life's enduring difficulties these families are going through. There is no turning back, we have to progress forward. We cannot do this with wavering thoughts, we need to pursue a plan that we can all follow and that will produce positive results. We need a plan that can motivate individuals, communities, and an entire nation to rise to greater self-achievements. The entire world is waiting and watching to see how South Africa escapes from their frustrated slow movement to progress. You have traveled now on a far journey with one intention of reaching a destination where people can live their lives without suffering from this disease whether or not they are rich or poor. You should not have to endure or live a painful life because you are infected with the H.I.V. virus. This mission we are on is to rid the world of this disease. Even if a cure should take a long time to be discovered, love and respect for our fellow brothers and sisters should be of high priority. Don't be afraid to talk about this disease; talking about it is part of the treatment process and the cure we currently have available. Having open communication about this disease is a measure of our success against it. As we move in this direction we stand to benefit greatly. This approach will help lead to a coordinate international approach to develop better strategies along with getting more scientific approaches available. A clear and sustainable approach will bring about a sense of urgency and commitment on the part of the international communities. HIV/AIDS maybe forgotten, but it is not cured; he have to take a stand and stand up and be educated and educate others about this disease.

In The New England Journal of Medicine, "Pediatric HIV-A Neglected Disease?" by Marc Lallemant, M.D., Shring Chang, Ph.D., Rachel Cohen, M.P.P., and Bernard Pecoul, M.D. M.P.H. N Engl J Med 2011; 365: 581 August 18, 2011.

According to this article, there is a global neglect when it comes to children; despite the overwhelming increase in the spread of HIV/AIDS, among children at birth, for various reasons: mothers not given antiretroviral medications during pregnancy, or failure to have medical attention during pregnancy. Serious attentions are not placed on this void. Researches have shown that early treatments do help, but little attention is paid to pediatric antiretroviral medications. It is frightening to identify the reasons why; when it is known that transmission of the HIV virus do occur during the birth process. Transmission of the HIV virus is preventable, and in wealthy countries primary efforts are made to preventing mother-to-child transmission.

When it comes to research for new intervention and treatments, to rid the world of this disease, the possibilities are endless. On the other hand, there seems to be a slow down when this include research for pediatric medications.

"Yet there is no such pipeline for pediatric HIV. Because it has been virtually eliminated in wealthy countries, pharmaceutical companies have little incentive to develop child-appropriate formulations. Children with HIV-AIDS in low-and middle –income countries are not considered in the HIV research and development agenda because they are poor and voiceless and do not represent a lucrative market in the traditional sense."

From early childhood to young adulthood can be a challenging time period; base on emotional, physical, social and psychosocial developmental adjustments. Challenges through these time periods can have life long consequences if not taken up and address their needs. Parents and young children need to be educated about their health which will enable them to become responsible participants in their lives. Growing up where both mother and father is dead can be a life long challenge.

With such potential neglect, we have to do everything possible to help children bypass these sequences of neglect. We have to start by educating the public, so they can educate their children, so this line of neglect can be subsided. From early childhood to young adulthood, can be a challenging time period for parents as well as children. This time period requires a delicate approach from both parents and children, but more so parents. As parents, we know of the potential dangers that lie ahead from a world that seems so innocent to the young minds. Challenges through these delicate time period, can have life long consequences.

According to American Academy Of Child & Adolescent Psychiatry, No. 62; May 2005, "Talking To Your Kids About Sex" "Talking to your children about love, intimacy, and sex is an important part of parenting. Parents can be very helpful by creating a comfortable atmosphere in which to talk to their children about these issues. However, many parents avoid or postpone the discussion."

Parents should not forget the difficult times they had talking about sex to their parents when they were growing up. I can remember how awkward it was to share how I was feeling. Time has changed, but that initial need to bond with an adult remains the same. Today children are more exposed to things we do want them to know and those we do not. As parents we have to develop strategies that will be of help to us and less stressful to the children. Remember, if we are not there to give them the correct information, miss guided information are there to mislead them.

Don't be a protector when it comes to your child, be an educator. They will be informed about the world out there, but don't be afraid, be one step ahead. From their early years, take them out to eat, games and to the movies. Use these opportunities to talk to your child about their bodies. Start by talking about their teeth; let them know that they have to keep their teeth clean because it will fall out one day and another one will come back. Let them know that their bodies will go through changes; some will be painful while others will be loving.

Not all children will have the same curiosity about their bodies. Others will be informed by older children. Develop a positive relationship with your child where they will not be afraid to let you know what is going on in their lives. As they grow older let them know of the important to talk about the responsibilities and consequences that come from being sexually active. Help them to understand that decision made today, has life long consequences. In talking to your child or adolescent, it is helpful to:

- Develop a close relationship with your child.

- Try to be a parent as well as a friend to your child.
- Talk to your child on a one to one basis; not a group.
- Obtain the level of knowledge your child has regarding sexual issues.
- Do not be ashamed to talk or answer questions about sex.
- Try to know what your child knows about sex.
- Read an age appropriate book that discusses sex.
- When a child asks about sexual matters, do not ignore the questions.
- Talk to your child about changes they are going to see in his/her body.

By allowing your child to fell comfortable to communicate with you about sexual matters, this will help open discussions about question you and your child may have to talk with each other about.

These are important steps in helping our children to be more informed about their bodies. Informing and communicating with our children will help them to protect themselves from those who will act inappropriately in a sexual, physical or emotional manner. This will give our children an outlet to inform parents or an outside adult that they feel uncomfortable with certain behavior an individual performs. We have to take a universal approach when it comes to protecting our children whether family member or an outsider. Enough problems are in the world today, we cannot allow our children to suffer emotional scars that they have to live with for the rest of their lives. Remember, we as adults have to put ourselves where they are when having sexual discussions. For a younger and sensitive child, make correlation with other subjects they are interesting in. Let them know that you do not have all the answers; you are in search of solutions. I remind you, the best screening is to make awareness sooner rather than later.

In an UpTodate article, "Management and Sequelae of Sexual abuse in Children and adolescents." Authors: Kirssten Bechtel, MD, Berkeley L. Bennett, MD, MS. Section Editors: Daniel M Lindberg, MD, Amy B Middleman, MD, MPH, MS ED, JAN E Drutz, MD. Deputy Editor: James F Wiley, II, MD, MPH. "INTRODUCTION-Sexual abuse occurs when a child engages in sexual activity for which he or she cannot give consent, is unprepared for developmentally, and cannot comprehend. This includes fondling and all forms of oral-genital, or anal contact with the child (whether the victim is clothed or unclothed), as well as non-touching abuses such as exhibitionism, or involving the child in pornography."

There are various changes and impacts a child undergoes when raped. A responsible adult must take immediate action to ensure emotional and physical stability o this child's well being. It is always encouraging to have a personal relationship with your child; this help the child to trust and communicate with you freely without being fearful of being blame. If passage of time should occur, it can be problematic physically as well as psychologically. Immediate attention needs to be taken. Seeking immediate medical attention where physical assessments needs to be done, while at the same time emotional care and getting legal assistance involvement.

Physical examination of the child could be challenging because it makes the child feels as if they are going through that assault all over. In such cases, knowledgeable professional needs to be involved. During such examination, it should be done in a way where it becomes part of the healing process. For example, the victim should be reassured and encouraged. The child is not the only one who needs help; members of the family may also need counseling. The child should never left to feel victimized again by uninformed family members. This will be a life long procession of giving reassurance and support to the victim.

Child molestations have been at the forefront; something that has been swept aside quietly. Regardless if the abusers are a family member, stranger or someone the family trusted with their children, these practices has to stop. What does this has to do with HIV/AIDS? It has everything to do with it. First, we have to do whatever possible to stop these relentless sexual abusers to stop inflicting life long tragedy on or children. On the other hand, we cannot afford to breed new generation of sexual abusers. These trends need to stop by us standing up against child sexual molesters.

In the face of impossbilities, caring parents and loving family members in South Africa feel as if they are alone in a crowded world. Where on earth do you have family member raping their own family member. This turmoil has to stop; and it begins with us the world communities. We will not stop until these shameful acts are made to be seen for their disgusting and inhumane behaviors.

The phrase "Legitimate Rape", was used by one politician, who shortly found out that rape is rape and there is nothing legitimate about that act. The same outrage goes for those who take advantage of our children. It may look far away when we read about family raping a four year old in South Africa, but we too have responsibility to safeguard our children.

In a New York Times article, "Who Would Abduct a Child? Previous Cases Offer Clues", by Mary Duenwald August 27, 2002. "Many abductors harbor sexual fantasies that involve children, and may exercise these fantasies by using child pornography. Many others pick on children only because they may be easier or more convenient, said Mark Hilts, a supervisory special agent for the F.B.I. who specializes in child abductions for the National Center for Analysis of Violence Crime. It is often said that abductors are people who themselves were abused as children."

It is frightening to see the number of children who are kidnapped each year. I am not here to frighten you or to make you become pessimistic about your child's where about. I am here to inform you and to allow you to be an eye and an ear for friends and families. The three young girls kidnapped in Cleveland over ten years is a prime example of getting lost and ignored. We all regretted what had happen to them, but at the back of our minds, we are still asking ourselves one questions. Why didn't I know? The young are the most vulnerable. Let us keep an open eye and ear for them. Report something looking or feeling suspicious to the authorities.

This article clearly gives us an insight that we are all vulnerable to these gruesome abuses. No matter where in the world children are, they subject to these sexual attacks. These perpetrators make our children subject to acquiring these deadly sexually transmitted diseases. No matter where we are, we have to defend our children. Like the statistics have shown us, an individual who was abused as a child has a greater propensity to become an abuser to a child.

Chapter 13

FREEDOM OF ASSAULTS AND
MEASURES OF PRIDE

W HILE SOUTH AFRICA GOES through their turmoil of sexual inappropriateness, the other parts of the world have their short comes also. Some of these hidden behaviors, if not exposed, they continue not to be spoken about. This include brothels all across the globe; this is where young girls are taken from their families and brought to perform and engage in sexual acts at an early age it is sad to read about these acts that often times taken as a right of passage. Ironically, there is nothing right about this. Mature grown men pay brothel owners to have sex with these young girls; and if not done, they are punished severely by any means necessary to show ownership and control over these innocent young girls. They are given nothing in return, whether financially or emotionally. Men are not required to wear protections while having sex with these girls. This often times leads to pregnancies, and or acquiring one or more of those deadly STD's (sexually transmitted disease.)

In the book, Half The Sky, by Nicholas D. Kristof and Sheryl WuDunn, tells of young girls taken to brothels or sex trading against their will in certain parts of the world. Some of these young girls are taken from a very young age to service men sexually at little to no financial incentive. In India, these girls are from lower economic caste with little to no education; ironically, girls from the upper class are not targeted. When you take a close look, you can see gender and social inequalities when it comes to sex slaves. These young girls pride are taken away from then from an early age and are left to the mercy of these sex shop owners. The greed of these brothel owners are driven by financial incentives, while ignoring the lives of innocent young girls. In many of these communities, the calls for help are often ignored. It often appears that the law enforcement in these communities make excuses for not fighting backs while these cruel acts continues. The living conditions these girls have to live under are horrible. These brothels are made of board shacks with dirt floor, in divided rooms. They are never allowed out of the premises. They are not allowed to use protection while having sex. Children of the sex workers are kept as a control method so the mothers faired to leave. Sometimes the sex workers are raped, beaten, and humiliated by the brothel owners.

I encouraged everyone to get a copy of this book, "Half The Sky", by Nicholas D. Krisstof and Sheryl WuDunn. This is a wonderful book with real life distresses and triumphs young girls go through as sex slaves. Seen what these young girls go through from a tender age of innocence taken away abruptly by older men and women to satisfy their financial aspirations. In doing so, these young girls loss hope of who they are and destroy any sense of hope. Their communities and society around them have no sympathy for these girls. Instead, from their lack of actions against these brothel owners, they also contributed. Societies need to rise up, rise up against these social intolerances and behaviors.

I take this time to wish Malala Yousafzai, fourteen year old girl from the town of Mingoro Swat District in the Pakistan, a complete recovery. She was shot a few days ago in October 2012 for speaking out against injustice against females and promoting equalities for all human beings. Though they tried to silence you, your voice is echoing across the globe. I encourage your determination to speak up for equality and against injustices. You have encouraged many other young people, to stand up for a better tomorrow. Speedy recovery, you have encouraged us; we encourage you, find your strength in love. The words from Whitney Houston's song, "Greatest Love of all"

I believe the children are our future

Teach them well and let them lead the way
Show them all the beauty they possess inside.

As human beings, we all have an internal drive that pushes us further than we recognize or can understand; I call this, measure of pride. This sense of awareness empowers one to transform that sense of weakness into self-awareness. This transformation, leads to self-empowerments that no one can take away from another person. Despite years of betrayals, mistreatments and discouragements, one moment of self-awareness, can help turn around the life of an abused person. Courage is an internal power, when put into action can change the dynamic of any given situation. When aspiration for hope is guided by perseverance, a mean for a better life can be achieved.

Women and children bare the brunt of most discriminations and inequalities on the face of this planet. We call young boys and young girls children. We cannot afford for them to grow up with animosity against each other. Young girls grow up to be women and young boys grow up to be men. We need to educate our children from an early age to distinguish the difference and value the strength between male and females and not to discriminate. We may never get to fully understand this phenomenon, but we are at a time and cross word in history where the world needs to change. This is not impossible. Women and young people need to be given the opportunity to contribute to society. This can be achieved through educating the population and providing jobs. We cannot keep one sector of society locked away. Unintelligent men try to control their surroundings by using one or all of the following tactics: intimidation, power or control. I am here to let the world know that this won't work any longer. A matter of fact, those who have been unprivileged are using these same tactics in a positive way to gain their freedom from abuses and neglects. We need the intelligence of men and women to work together for a better future. Given the plight of female in societies around the world, we have a lot to learn. I believe a revolution is coming, unlike none we have seen before. Why do I say this? Well, if you consider women to be the enemy, they are living with us, raising our children, cooking our meals, giving us emotional support; women are doing all this without fussing. Women know what to do; we just need to love and encourage women, so doubts and fear do not hinder their aspirations.

The soft voice and tender foot steps of Mahatma Gandhi drove India to their freedom. This one preacher, had a dream, Doctor Martin Luther King Jr., his dream led to the rebirth of a nation. Rosa Parks, did not go to the back of the bus, she stood firm on what she believed in. Oprah Winfrey, she had a rough childhood, yet she rise above it; today she is one of the richest and influential women helping young girls all across the world. Harriet Tubman, a black woman who could not read, yet she led the path of the underground railroad for many to receive freedom from slavery. Mother Teresa was born in Albania, citizen of India. She stood firm for equal justice and recognition of the poor. Her love had no limits for the needy and those suffering. Princess Diana, cared for the sick, healthy, blacks, whites; it did not matter what race you were to her. She was a princess for the world. I was amaze to see some of the places she visited; yet she did without any second guessing. Her death was tragic, yet here we are today writing about how influential her presence was while she was alive. President Nelson Mandela spent many years in a prison, in his own country for taking a stand for justice and freedom. Truth and justice rains with the constant reminder of injustices under Apartheid rule; not long after getting out of prison Mr. Nelson Mandela was elected president of South Africa. President Ronald Ragan of the United States of America demanded President Mikhail Gorbachev of the Soviet Union to tear the walls down that separated East and West Germany. Before President Mikhail Gorbachev could have responded, the people of East and West Germany were shaking each other hands with no barriers separating them. I too have a dream that men and women will love and respect each other. This love will transcend through the homes out into the communities. The battle has started and we will not stop until each nation rise up to the responsibility of protecting their citizen, from the unborn to the elderly. We can and we have to do better. We have to protect women and young girls from these torturous and inhumane acts. We believe in love, one for another; you may not see it, but it is there waiting for you. I believe that each success can lead to another challenge that we will eventually overcome. When it comes to human rights, economic opportunities, reproductive rights, educational empowerments, women are looked at differently from men. Given a chance for a better world, men and women have to work with each other. Lets put aside: discrimination, sexism, raping, mental and physical abuse; a better world exist when we can work with each other. This has been a journey of hope and restoration for men and women around the globe. Words from the song of Michael Jackson, "Man in the Mirror", I'm Gonna Make A Change, For Once In My Life.

Chapter 14

EDUCATING THE PUBLIC ABOUT HIV

H IV IS KNOWN AS the Human immunodeficiency virus; a virus that attacks white blood cells called helper T cells (CD4) and reduces their fighting capacity to a low level. These cells are part of the immune system which helps fight against infections. They fight off infections and diseases. Being exposed to the HIV virus lets one become vulnerable to diseases the body would naturally fight. Diagnosis of HIV can be done through blood test or saliva. Most time, the blood test is done to confirm an accurate result. Early infection may show a false negative result. A person may need to wait a few weeks in order for the correct result to be identified. Medical labs have different ways of obtaining the correct result. Early symptoms may include fever that does not go away, muscle weakness, diarrhea, and swollen lymph glands. Immediate medical attention is needed; his person needs to be seen by a medical doctor.

Here you will be given a full medical examination and with questions and answers. Base on your symptoms and answers, a variety of tests will need to be done. This will include tests for the HIV virus. During the early stage of an HIV infection, you do not have AIDS, which I will explain later. Treatments will be given to subside your symptoms; it may include hospitalization for a few days.

AIDS is a late stage of HIV infection, which includes the destruction of T cells or CD 4 counts. At this point the body is unable to fight against infection, signaling a severe insult to the immune system. Treatments need to be started once a person has a confirmed positive HIV test. This is to prevent one's immune system from further insults. There is no cure for HIV/AIDS currently, only treatments to prevent illnesses from this disease. These treatments are called antiretroviral drugs. While taking these treatments, the virus can still be transmitted to another person. These medication prevents the virus from multiplying.

The HIV virus is spread trough contact with HIV contaminated blood or other body fluids which may include semen, vaginal fluid, or breast milk.

Here is something I want to talk about. We need to develop a plan people can use to fight against this disease and its unwelcome affects. Since there is no cure at the present time, only medications can decrease the viral load in the body, I believe we have to do something to decrease the spread of this disease.

We have to focus on: Identification of the Problem, develop conflict resolution, review of modifications process. For example, we have identified raping of young children as a problem. Now we need to develop resolution that will combat this problem. Educating the communities about the HIV virus and how this virus is transmitted and the illness it produces. We also need to educate both young and old people on the function of the human body. We also need to communicate the devastated emotional effect raping young children causes. Developing potential modification may include having sociologists and psychologists talk to the communities about encouraging behaviors that promotes human growth and development. Increase the presence of the police in the communities; this will generate a sense of safety and calm. Have religious and political leaders have frequent meetings in the communities; this will give a sense of reassurance that the community is not left along. The judicial system should be firm on these criminals. Increased social pressures on these criminal offenders where they cannot be comfortable. There are many other issues that we can use this model to help resolved, from financial deficits in the family, social isolations, depression, fatigue, and malnutrition families are going through because the bread winner in the family dies or maybe children are left to take care of children. Reviewing potential modifications may include criminals doing community services under close observation so other may be deterred from doing or getting involved in some inappropriate behaviors.

This is also helpful for criminals to get reformed and become aware of promoting and contributing to society, instead of eroding social norms. This will help young people to see the contribution they can make to promote a better tomorrow. It is better contributing to the growth of society where you are free rather than being locked up in prison. Other potential modifications may also include having conferences with different social group so open dialogues and exchange of information can help ease misinformation about antisocial behaviors. This model is only one way of helping to educate people of all ages about each other. There are other approaches we can look at. At the presence, we need a plan that can be implemented by the common person to the government of a nation. We cannot take the simplest of ideas for granted, something need to be done right away. We have to be smarter than our past and be ready for the future.

Our model of care needs to be a confidence builder. At first many may not understand how to implement different measures of this plan, but with supportive proponents we can see improvement. There should be no debate over this strategy. Instead we should allow time to be spent so we can get a fair evaluation of this model. Failure to give a good assessment could lead us to slow down or set backs. We have to be persistent in our drive to awaken the awareness of people all around and be there to support people as they persist through these difficult times. The determination to succeed will be strongly dependent on outside support and our internal desire for change. Following this model will allow us to see if there is a reduction in the spread of HIV Virus, increase in education of the community on all frontiers, increase in government support for community programs, government enhance the safety of the communities, food distribution centers, increase in medical services to the communities, stress reduction centers where counselors are available, decrease to elimination of child raping, increase in adoption of children, and maybe development of group homes for young children. There are many other things to be done; including the global community suffering from the HIV/AIDS epidemic could benefit from these interventions. We will not force individuals to make choices, however, I have a self-consciousness to help educate people around the world how they can live healthier and have reduction in preventable diseases. I support governments who support the need for their citizens to achieve and maintain good health by providing essential health care, medical supplies and services in order to improve their quality of life.

To help support the different communities, we have to subdivide the communities in a manner where they will be supported and encouraged. As we develop stronger support groups, we will better have identifiable markers that can be evaluated. We need to look at service, quality of improvement, and growth. The service provided need to be one that promotes love, compassion and empathy. Majority of the people will be trying to live with the effects of this disease while at the same time being a strong pillar for the community. There will need to be improvement in services provided. The symptoms of this disease can be from dehydration due to diarrhea to memory loss. There need to be a quick response to help someone going through these symptoms. Improvement in the quality of medical care to public safety by the police and law enforcement need to be addressed. The communities must be able to identify places where services can be accessed in a fast and efficient manner. We can no longer have six feet by six feet H.I.V. testing site centers where majority of the people in the community need to be tested. With growth, emphasis has to be placed on means of services where people will feel empowered and supported. With improvement in services more people should seek care for themselves. With greater outreach to the communities, people will believe in themselves more and promote healthier ways of living.

In the immediate presence of this catastrophe, we have to find ways to escape from further disasters. People all over the world need help. I am not just talking about one region in the world; this is a global problem requiring global response. We are not confined to one region of the world, we are mobile and transparent. Here where we stand, the struggle against this disease goes on. Antiretroviral drugs are great life savers, but they are not cures. Both young and older people are potential carriers of this deadly virus; we cannot ignore this fact. We have to carry on a global education and outreach to combat the bad effects this disease has done. As you have seen, the battle is on multiple fronts. There are cultural misconceptions that need to be overcome; we cannot accept the belief that having sex with virgins will result in cure from this disease. This crisis is no excuse to ignore the entire social and economic set backs of your country. You need to implement meaningful ways that will encourage the people to be more informed about their health rather than watching them perish. We can start by educating the public by giving them the right information. We are all vulnerable to this disease and must be made aware of things we can do, especially teenagers and young adults. We will take a look at informing teenagers and the older adults about HIV.

In the article, UpToDate, "Patient information: Adolescent sexuality", written by author Paul AS Benson, MD, MPH, Section Editor Amy B Middleman, MD, MPH, MS & Deputy Editor Mary M Torchia, MD. "Sexual development is an important part of health, similar to other measures of physical growth, such as height and weight. Sexual behavior, which is related to sexual development, has important health implications for everyone, and especially for teens. It is particularly important that teens be well informed about all aspects of sex and sexual health."

On the caravan of love, actions taken, elevates our pursuit for meaningful actions. Across the globe, we read about the millions of people dying and being infected by the HIV virus. We are in the third decade of this battle. I believe we have to inform the world about this deadly plague. It appears that over the years some elected officials have done little or even ignored the impact this epidemic has had on their population. Young people, you are the future leaders and citizens of this world. You can make a change for the better. We are a sexual being for pleasure or procreation. Sharing love with another human being should not be rewarded with illness or death. I believe the more we get to know ourselves, the more we are able to make important decisions about our sexuality.

Human sexuality is complex and dynamic. There are many ways to acquire the HIV virus, but I believed the majority of exposure to this disease was through sexual contacts. In other words, we share our bodies with other humans because we are a loving species. On every living continent across the globe, we have significant exposure to this disease.

At an appropriate age parents or guardians of children needs to proactive and inform them about changes they will experience in their bodies. As a child becomes older, certain hormonal changes will occur in their bodies. These changes will leads to different development changes for each gender. For females you will have breast development, facial hair in boys, and growth of hair under the arms and in the genital area of both boys and girls.

As ones body develops, you often have a desire to be intimate sexually. Such desires are normal, but needs to be implemented wisely. Many factors need to be taken into consideration such as: early pregnancy, financial responsibility of taking care of a child, and acquiring sexually transmitted diseases. This is a turmoil time in a teenager's life. While the focus is on the HIV virus, there are many other sexually transmitted diseases that need the outlook. Benign neglects are no excuses; most times, once infected, you remain infected for life.

Human sexuality starts from an early age and develops throughout the life cycle. I will now look at the need of the older adult. On the website UpToDAte.com, "HIV and the older Patient" wrote by Aurthors Charulata Jain Sabharwal, MD, MPH. Nathalie Casau-Casau-Schulhof, MD. Section Editor John G Bartett, MD. Deputy Editor Barbara H McGovern, MD. "With the introduction of more potent therapies, a greater prevalence of HIV-infected individuals over the age of 50 is projected over the next decade. This epidemiologic trend is expected due to longer survival of HIV-infected patients on antiretroviral therapy, and to increased case finding due to wider HIV testing. HIV infection in the older patient is associated with delays in diagnosis due to unsuspected HIV infection, age-related differences in immune responses to HIV antigens." The spread of the HIV virus and reported AIDS cases in adults aged 50 years or older has increased. HIV testing in the older adults is population has often done at a slower rate for unknown reasons; this failure often leads to progression of the disease because treatments started late. Older adults are involved in sexual activities just like younger adults. Because most times, older adults are given the benefits of the doubts, their sexual partners ignored believing that they can be infected with an STD. We have to wake up, acquiring STD's does not have age limitations. We can no longer look at someone and suggest that they are HIV positive like the early years. Today you cannot tell the infected from the uninfected.

Male and female have a different approach to their sexuality. Some females look at sex as a sacred act, while most male look at it as an activity that needs to be done and moved on. I believe that because so much of the female sexual organs are internal and need to be protected, females have a different view when it comes to their sexuality. This cannot be taught, I believe it is instinctual for females' protection regarding sex. To the male, his sexual organs are external where not a lot of protection is needed, so he behaves as such. This mentality is deep.

Looking at the younger adults and older adults, both of them have a sense of vulnerability to this disease HIV, as well as other STD's. Younger adults are driven by the need to explore, while the older adults are set in their mind that they are beyond being infected with these STDs. With this mind set, more education needs to be done in our society. We are all vulnerable to these diseases, and must do everything we can to reduce our vulnerability. With the discoveries of medications for men with erectile dysfunction, more and older men are engaging in risky sexual activities with sexual partners that engage in loose sexual relationships. Behaviors such as these put the older men at a higher risk for acquiring sexual diseases. If the older man was HIV positive, using medications to correct erectile dysfunction, now gives him a renewed energy to engage in sexual activities. Such behavior leaves the entire family at risk and vulnerable. Most times the older men will try to engage a younger female into sexual acts; this act leaves a spiraling defeat to the family structure. If the male is married, then he leaves a vulnerable wife at home to the possibilities of acquiring a sexually transmitted disease. If the older male is single, he now leaves a young female into a family structure that often times are not functional; she is left alone to raise a family. I have nothing against producer of medications to help men with erectile dysfunction; I am just saddened that more education is not given to the public about the risks of acquiring sexually transmitted diseases from a younger or older person base on their sexual behaviors. Manufactures of these medications that help men regain their sexual vigor, should also be responsible for educating the public of the short and long term effects of these medications when it comes to men's sexual behaviors.

There is no end to this call. The caravan of love trail needs you to be an active member. There is so much to be done. With more help the call for assistance won't go unanswered. Encouraged a friend, talk to someone about this call. The goal of this movement is to move victims of this disaster from being victims to leaders. Doing this shows the world that we love and care about each other. We wont allow desperate or foolish acts to bring set backs to our goal. Join the caravan of love trail today. We start with the government of South Africa, with effective governance things can improve. This will allow the international communities to join together and local communities to overlook the slow movements of progress. There need to be a transition from the old way of thinking to a more dynamic way of pursuing a better approach. This will allow us to achieve measurable progress that will bring about improvement in the lives of many. We need clear and sustainable approaches in order to achieve short and long term successes. The weight of this crisis will not determine the future of South Africa, nor any other country going through this crisis with the HIV epidemic; let it be known, help is on the way. I appreciate the world's approach to this crisis, though in some cases we have been very slow. The new awakening is upon us. We cannot ignore this call for help. There are things that should never be attempted, such as attempting to empty the ocean with a tea spoon; this is an impossible task. However when you have the power to fix it, fix it and don't sweat it; let God take care of impossibilities. Let us do the best we can with whatever resources we have. Live happy for yourself and others around you; feed your body, soul and spirit with encouragements releasing endless opportunities in motion, for the eyes to see and for us to achieve a better future.

You have journeyed with us on this far journey and now discovered something about yourself. Maybe never before in your life, you thought you could tolerate such a vast experience, but you have. You did not give up. You will not allow others around you to quit. You are a resourceful entity on this journey of love. Along this long journey, you asked for little, because everything you needed you have inside of you. You comforted me, making this journey as relaxing as possible. Traveling on the caravan of love has brought up issues of the past that still lingers around, yet we did not allow them to derail our journey. Tell me what have you learned? I have learned that the human spirit is a strong force to isolate. We do not give up easy even on the last lap on this journey of life. The human spirit will rise above all set backs and prove there is a greater purpose for living. We will one day find a cure for this disease and many others. We will no longer be afraid to share ourselves with each other out of love. The greater forces of love will confined those that take advantages of this weakness.

I remember driving to school in 1991 when I heard the news flash, Magic Johnson of the LA Lakers has the HIV virus. I can never forget that day. I loved him as a player, he was one of my heroes that motivated me to do the right things in life, his passion for the game of basketball transcend across the globe. The deep question I had at the time, why him? I did not have an answer. When I watched that news conference, I felt angry, betrayed, out of place and puzzled. A sense of denial and disbelief was over me. I felt this way at the time because something like this should not happen to a person like Magic Johnson. In my mind, getting the HIV virus only occurred to drug users or people who engaged in careless sexual behaviors. I confess, this belief was a misconception on my part. From that news conference; I changed my outlook on human sexuality. There was a sense of unknown about who to trust at this time. Many people found it difficult to understand why we were all so vulnerable to this disease.

At the time, obtaining the HIV virus was like a death sentence. According to Magic Johnson, "A part of my life is gone." There was a great level of ignorance about having the HIV virus. At the news conference he announced his retirement from the game of basketball; after a year he came back, but it did not last for long. Many players did not want to play on the basketball court with Magic. To see a player like Magic Johnson go through such turmoil was humiliation, makes me and many others sad. Over the years I have lived a life courteous of this disease; neither myself, anyone in my family or any friends of mine have this disease. Why am I so active in this cause? I am a person who cares about others.

Not very far from sexual abuse of children is sexual discrimination of adults who are HIV positive or has AIDS. Sexual abuse of children and sexual discrimination of adults cannot be placed in the same categories; however, they both have their own legal ramifications. For some adults infected with the HIV virus, experience emotional, psychological, laughter, neglects and abuses. These discriminatory behaviors exist in society where it makes being HIV positive a disgrace. Regardless of how one acquired this virus, no one should be abused or discriminated against. The caravan of love is an alliance forge with bravery, hope for mankind and justice for all.

Chapter 15

CALLED TO ACTION

MY DESTINY ON THIS trip was fulfilled when I went to Ghost Mountain, in South Africa. There it was confirmed that I had a great part to play in fulfilling helping many people to escape from the suffering of this disease. I accept this responsibility and have become a crusader in fighting against this disease. This journey has taught me a lot. It takes a lot more energy to overcome something bad than it does for doing something good. Therefore I encourage us to continue fighting for the good of mankind. Time and distance has reached a common ground where they exist together. This is our moment for all eyes to see. You cannot escape or hide from me. The journey was long, but we endured. Get up my brother, get up my sister, it's not over yet. When you give and try all you can and feel like giving up, here I stand. Time and distance will have a common ground. No need to look back; all you would see is the dust that I have shaken off. Rise up my brother, rise up my sister. The sun is shining forth on a new day. The night cannot escape the light of the moon. Wherever I go, there is enough light for me to see; all around me is full with love.

I am a caravan and I am strong. There is no limit to the amount of load I can carry. I am a caravan that does not sleep or require those that join me to loose their cheer. I am a caravan that will not stop or procrastinate for one moment. I will ignore the thoughts of those that encourage my demise. I will never empty my load nor can I ever be filled up. There are no numbers to my existence or time for my demise.

There is one thing that I am full of and that is love. You can enter being empty, but guarantee to be filled up in a short while. I do not encourage you to forget where you are coming from; just remember we are on this journey of love together. It is your responsibility to take along others with you, on this sense of never ending love. No one is a second class citizen on the caravan of love journey. We all are equal in each others sight. This is important so that no one will be allowed to create a moment of inferiority complex against the others. There will be no time to make someone else fall off this wagon. If you are fill with doubts, clouded with uncertainties you have a lot to learn. You may have come aboard with skepticism, but very soon you will be overcome with relentless love and enthusiasm. You cannot overcome this force; you will have to give in to a soaring positive empowerment. Be not afraid, you are traveling on the caravan of love. You won't have to pay a price for this encounter, only avail yourself to journey on the caravan of love that you will never forget. One of the pursuits of this journey is to overcome negative behaviors. You won't be surprised to put away all the negative forces and to extend yourself to claim the entire positive end you can claim. There are no limitations to achieve positive goals. No matter what short come there might be, you are now rested on the caravan of love. When you look around at others and see that you are no different, then this should give you a push to achieve more than what was presented to you.

I have learned that the HIV/AIDS epidemic is frightening, painful, devastating experience that leads to unimaginable chaos in one's life. However, there is one thing I know for my personal life and existence and that of others is that death is expected on this journey. Life comes along with challenges and mysteries that makes the expected welcoming; this welcome comes to free the suffering and the under privileged. The mysteries of our existence make life meaningful, graceful, challenging and puzzling. What we learn from each experience we face makes us better equipped to face the difficult challenges lies unseen. Some of the most precious resources we have not yet founded. Life's challenges push us to that point that makes us better individuals, equipped to deal with new challenges. For each day we live, each day that passes by; we draw closer to accepting that final phase of our existence. The mysteries and challenges that come during those other days will bring about joy, pain, suffering and love. It is up to us to master these feelings that accompany us on this journey. Something would be wrong if only one of these emotions accompanies us. We have to learn to accept them all and allowing a small percentage of them all to coexist with us. We have to rise to the occasion of learning how to manipulate and filter these emotions. Remember, death is expected only once, but life's journey poses many challenges and chances where life's occurrences can occur as many time as possible.

Even though death occurs once, before its arrival the sufferings life brings, sometimes seems more stagnant and painful than we can bear. We looked at the arrival of death as an escape from the physical, emotional, psychological and spiritual pain we must bear. Once death gets here, it also relieves us humans of many unbearable sufferings we once had to endure. We have to learn to incorporate death into our daily lives, so boundaries will be torn away so family members can have a calmer transitions and go on living their lives more meaningfully after the death of a love one. This is one way of developing a winning outlook on this disease. This disease process can affect and make us prone to many illnesses, despite all the sufferings one goes through. The final outcome can be prepared for in advance.

The persons who are infected should not isolate themselves from the public or their families. A winning and positive approach needs to be taken allowing others to take an encouraging approach to helping them adjust to this disease that will allow you to live and enjoy life to its fullest in the face of death. There is no doubt that death will be part of our experience whether we have a healthy or an unhealthy physical condition. As much as we plan for tomorrow, we should also have a plan and be prepared for death. Unfortunately, in some circumstances the death of a family member or a close friend brings this realization front and center. It is unfortunate, but most of the focus should be on a person while they were alive, not while they are dead. This approach will help bring about closure and acceptance of the passing of a love one which will bring about healing. This book is not only about the plight and suffering of innocent people, but it is about us. We are all human beings. Sometimes it is puzzling to me why someone had to suffer while I am free of those short comes. For the things we can do in life to make ourselves healthy, we should do them and stay away from unhealthy lifestyles. This is personal for everyone; some people engage in unsafe behaviors, and others engage in risky behaviors.

While you may not engage in risky sexual behaviors, you may be someone who has an unhealthy drinking habit. You might have been raped and contracted some deadly STD's. You may have had a night out and had a little to drink and taken advantage of. You may have given your heart to someone you thought loved you and in so shared your body with someone who did not tell you they were HIV positive. Do not be ashamed; it was not your fault you became a victim. Remember; do not give up on love. Love would not have betrayed you or take advantage of your innocence. I give you love and hope that you and many others will not be forgotten. We are all on this planet together; we can make it better by seeking to do good things. Below listed is a model designed to help the care giver as well as those who are sick and are in need of help. This model helped to reduce frustration in a delicate environment where both the sick person and the care giver need to be in a therapeutic caring environment. This model will help the HIV infected person to accept that he/she is infected and will go about seeking medical assistance without being resentful to people around or shut him or herself away.

Chapter 16

DISCUSSING END OF LIFE ISSUES

INITIALLY, SOMETHING WILL DRIVE an individual to seek medical assistance because they feel something is wrong with their health. This could be the appearance of one of the signs and symptoms explained earlier. Taking that first step to seek medical assistance can be frightening. One can goes into depression waiting on a blood result. With a positive and confirmed HIV blood result, medical treatments will need to be started quickly. Along with medical treatments, psychological treatments will also need to be initiated Discussion on end of life's issues with a family member or a friend needs to be part of one's medical treatment plan failure to incorporate such discussion may lead to medical set backs for an individual.

This discussion can start by accepting your illness, while not blaming yourself. You may need to talk with your doctor first, who can encourage you and referred you to a professional who can further assist you with your decisions. You may find yourself going through changes that you yourself may not understand. You may be a family member who has lost someone due to HIV/AIDS; during their illness or after their death, you may need professional assistance. You may be someone who provides assistance to those with the HIV virus; you need assistance providing assistance to those in need. It may seem simple, but providing care for someone with a terminal illness is not easy. You think of yourself, your family and friends. I encourage you to treat everyone fairly.

You can start by understanding that the individual will be loaded with denial, frustration, anger, sadness, and feeling of ending their life. During time such as this, individuals needs to seek assistance from family or friends and dig deep within themselves for their own strengths and develop healthy behaviors that will help them to regain their motivation.

Being HIV positive is not the end; yes you may be in a position where health care is not assessable like other places. Remember, whether here or wherever you may be, believe in yourself. What you may be going through is real, but help is on the way. The world is wringing a bell at the present moment. Some will hear it, other will ignore it. Trust me; this will not go on forever. Help is on the way.

All around the globe, this virus has infected and kill so many. A lot has been done, but it is still not enough. You are not alone; many more await help, but sadly left alone. The cry of the innocent waits to be answered.

The grieving process impacts all domains of an individual. You may find yourself unable to eat, go out and shop, you may even stop communicating with those around you. Time heals all wounds and broken hearts. Take time to seek help and talk about how you feel. Don't hide away, call someone and say something. Revenge on someone for what had happen to you served no purpose; it further diminish who you are.

The caravan of love tour is never ending. This path is for all of us who seek to find an enduring path that will not fail. When we take time to care for another person who has set backs or short comes in this life, it makes the world a better place. There will always be problems in this world. However, we do not have to be afraid or worry ourselves, because together we will work to solve these problems. Every spring we will change the clocks on our walls turning the clocks one hour ahead and in the fall do the opposite, turning the clocks one hour backwards. The fact of the matter is time remains the same; we are the one doing the adjusting. Time is a journey that has been, and will be regardless of the path we take. Let's make a path so bright that time itself will be amaze. We do this by loving each other. If we do this, time itself will be non existence. We will not wait on time to send a care package to someone over sea. With the present rules, if a government does not have diplomatic ties with another, then the relationship between the two countries is non existent. On the caravan of love, we will listen to soft or loud cries, crying out for help. It may seem impossible today that certain borders will not allow us to cross over.   But it is only a matter of time before that insurmountable mountain will become rubble of words lost in the past. We inject hope into the lives of those individuals who might feel lost in a world they do not know how it comes about. The crippling thing about fear is that it is not real; however, it can have an affect on the weak or strong where everything seems impossible to accomplish. We take a stand to acknowledge the lives of those individuals who fell victims to this disease. You are not forgotten. Your lives might of cut short, but the legacy you left behind will help fuel this ship to travel around the globe for restoration and regeneration, letting people know that they are victims and they should not victimize themselves. The exceptional lives they have lived will be remembered.

Chapter 17

CONTEMPORARY APPROACH

THE HUMAN MIND IS an exceptional instrument, used positively it can be a marvelous tool in aiding our daily walk and experiences. I had no fear going to South Africa because I knew the different modes of transmission for this disease; instead I got to learn a lot about the people suffering from this deadly disease and also myself. As long as I can remember, every morning I woke up, I usually woke up with an erection. This is due to hormonal changes that occur in the body at a certain; this happen to most healthy males. This was one way my body ensures me that my manhood was healthy, and my physical body was healthy. Because of this, every morning I went into the bathroom, I had to be very careful when I go to urinate, or else I would make a mess on and around the toilet. This was a little way of my body saying hello good morning to me when I woke up each morning. For the entire time I spent in South Africa, I did not have an erection whether it was morning, noon or night. My body went into a biological shut down; I believed this happened to ensure its safety. Unconsciously my mind was focusing on its normal sexual function as a detrimental passage; to prevent me from going down this path way, my body had a protective measure. I did not go to South Africa to have any sexual conquest; yet my body was thrown into a protective mode. I called what I went through SIPA; (Self Induced Penile Amnesia). I cherish this protective nature of the body's protective nature; so fragile yet so protective in its survival. It is ironic that so many of us take for granted or maybe ignored this delicate nature the human body used to protect us from danger. The time I spent in South Africa has been and continues to be a learning experience for me. Before going to South Africa, in my personal walk I practice SEPA when driven by internal emotions of grandeur. What I have just mentioned about practicing SEPA is personal and I did not have to let it be known. However, as men we need to take control of our sexual behaviors and settle down.

The next segment of this book will explain to you why I revealed this about myself. In the midst of any crisis, we need leaders who are strong, someone who will be a leader for the people and to the people. Someone who is not two faces; say one thing now and do the opposite behind close door. The people of South Africa have been through too much from past and current political leaders. Despite being overwhelmed by this crisis, they do not need to be taken advantage of.

Chapter 18

LIMITED LOVE CAPACITY?

I WAS IMPRESSED AT first when I read about the current president of South Africa; Mr. Jacob G. Zuma; who spoke on the direction he would like to see the country go when it comes to fighting HIV/AIDS. This was a total opposite approach from the previous administration ran by President Theodore Mbeki. I particular admired him for being bold and upfront on putting priority on the fight against HIV/AIDS, and allowing antiviral drugs to be part of this treatment process. It made me looked at him as a welcome leader despite being a foreigner looking in from the outside. However, as President Zuma spend more and more time under the spotlight as leader of his country, more personal and social revelation began to be exposed about him. These accusations began to show a two face leader, leading a country with desperate need of leadership and accountability.

In the beginning of his administration, we heard the words of a man that so many believed and trusted. From the New York Times article written by Celia W. Dugger, "Breaking With The Past, South Africa Issues Broad AIDS Policy" "Mr. Zuma announced that drug therapy for HIV.-positive pregnant women and babies would broaden and start earlier, and that HIV. Patient with tuberculosis would be treated earlier, while their immune systems are stronger. Both steps meshed new guidelines from the World Health Organization. Researchers have estimated that delays in providing drugs under Mr. Mbeki cost the lives of 35,000 babies and led to 330,000 premature deaths."

You can hear and feel the need for an urgent approach or care for people suffering from this devastating disease. The approach President Zuma took need to be respected giving great hope to those suffering from this deadly disease. The leader of a country is only one person, but emphasis they place on certain priorities, can change a country's outlook on whatever difficulties they are going through. I certainly felt President Zuma's approach to the HIV/AIDS epidemic was a welcoming approach starting his presidency with such a welcome approach. Unfortunately, not long into his presidency, a lot of Mr. Zuma's pass began to appear in the public, giving doubt to where he stand as a leader of this suffering nation.

According to the New York Times article, "South Africa: Zuma Acknowledges Paternity", by Barry Bearak Feb. 3, 2010. "President Jacob Zuma admitted Wednesday that he was the father of a girl born last October. Mr. Zuma, a polygamist, has three wives, but this baby was born out of wedlock, and allegations that the president had fathered 20th child have preoccupied the news media in South Africa since the story broke on Sunday. The country has one of the world's worst HIV. Infection rates and Mr. Zuma was criticized for undermining his own government's campaign against unprotected sex and multiple partners."

Immediately after it was published, President Zuma came out against those in the news media that made it known that he was the father of a baby girl outside of his marriages. I remind you, this is not a Shakespeare's tragedy, even though it does look to be one. Mr. Zuma is the president of his nation that is under going so much difficulty implementing the correct proposal to fight against this deadly disease. President Zuma criticized the news media, but he should be ashamed. It sent a conflicting report to the public, in what to believe. Behaviors such as this gave more strength to those rapists. This made the public keep waiting for an answer; an answer of whom to trust, who to guide them, and who to allow to comfort them. This may not be part of the thinking process of President Zuma, but this is how a leader should think before acting. Don't get me wrong, Mr. Zuma has his private life to live, but he is a public figure sending out confusing messages.

Chapter 19

A New Beginning!

I ENCOURAGE EVERYONE WHO has had painful moments in the past to develop strategies to make living life easier for their present. We sometime lost trust in those around us we looked up to. Unfortunately, they too need a moment for themselves to regain and identify who they are. This is the caravan of love, we leave no one behind. Mr. Zuma you are in a position to educate your country, be a motivating force so others will be encouraged to move ahead, help to attract people who will want to do better and help young people to be more mature. Help the youth of tomorrow to realize the power that is bestowed upon them. We have no one to blame than ourselves for neglecting to bestow the mantel of hard work upon the younger generation. The measure of our successes may not be seen for years or may not be able to be measured with techniques we have available today. However, we should not stop trying to make the future better for ourselves as well as for the future generations. I can understand the level of frustration we may have from the slow movements of progress on fighting the HIV/AIDS epidemic. We all like to see clear and sustainable growth in the decline of spreading of this virus. We all stand to benefit clearly from this progression; however, it is not easy. Sometimes we fail to see or realize the path our resolution and mechanism of change is going. Failure to adopt quickly sometimes pushes us farther back making us have to spend more time going over what we already have been through.

Effective and powerful ideologies should always be flexible to changes so adjustments can be made quickly. Failure to adjust quickly often times leads to chaos and loss of faith by those who need it most. When something like this happen, we often time has to start over; this end up costing more financially as well as loosing lives. We need clear and sustainable approaches that will pull communities together; not only local communities, but most of all the entire international communities. Some countries call this game football other calls it soccer. It is one game that draws the world communities together. This game was recently played in South Africa; the world cup. We united around playing for a world champion every four years. We cannot afford to wait another four years for the world community to come together against the spread of this disease. It does not matter by what method we go about calling the world's attention to this disease, it has to be done. We thank present and past world leaders who find it in their hearts to make a pledge to fight this disease. We are thankful for those who are deeply committed, yet they are so much more to be done. We all have new challenges with no single formula for resolutions. We must be seen as working together, and embrace the need to sour for unlimited human boundaries in the pursuit for providing aid for those that are sick and finding a cure for this disease. The mission of the caravan of love is to give people hope, helped to open doors of opportunities, bring peace and comfort to people's lives.

In a New York Times article, "South Africa Expand AIDS Treatments-Zuma." by Reuters December 1, 2009. PRETORIA (Reuters) - South Africa, which has the world's highest HIV caseload, will roll out life-prolonging anti-retroviral drugs to significantly more people infected with the virus from next year, President Jacob Zuma said on Tuesday. Zuma announced a new era in the approach to AIDS in South Africa, where at least 5.7 million people are infected with HIV and predecessor Thabo Mbeki was accused of failing to address a sickness that kills an estimated 1,000 people a day. "Let there be no ore shame, no more blame, about HIV and AIDS stop," Zuma said in a speech on World AIDS Day."

The previous president, President Mbeki's health ministers recommended garlic and beetroot as treatment for people infected with the HIV virus. It is now time for something to be done. Treatment of infected mothers and those with CD4 counts less than 350 is a good idea. Failure of a leader to react during a crisis, will only lead to disaster in the future. I applaud President Zuma for taking such bold steps in fighting against this disease. It was not easy, but this was the right thing to do. These implementations would take steps shortly, to those who are HIV positive.

The past two news paper articles give us the perspective of the difficult choices world leaders have to make. We can see the difficult choices of promises versus commitments. Though world leaders have HIV/AIDS as strong medical issues, South Africa is drawn to make more immediate proposals and plans due to many years of neglect and ignorance. The United States of America has a lot to gain and loose from their proposals of financial contributions to this cause. The world looks at America as a leader and proactive fighter against this disease. We already have seen on papers the financial cut backs that have been made to the fight against this disease. It may be seen as if the infected ones are left to fight this disease by themselves; however, it is not so.

In the midst of doors closing around, we need to stand up and show our resilience. We need to make loud noises so the world can hear us. We are fighting a war against WMDD. The vuvuzalas might have been making annoying sound at the world's cup, but we have to remain persistent and committed to what ever your cause may be about. The plan of the United States to scale back more HIV infected on drugs and to emphasize prevention is a shortcut on the fight against this disease. We are fighting a war that need an all out approach to claim victory. We all need an invitation to take better care of ourselves because the world cannot do it alone for us. I invite you to take care of yourself if you are not HIV positive. If you are HIV positive, I also invite you to believe in yourself knowing that you did not do this to yourself. Do not be revengeful and get someone infected intentionally. You are part of the human race that strives to live above our circumstances and will not allow yesterday to curve a path for our tomorrow. Let us focus on our here and now.

The caravan of love focuses way beyond our sorrows and misfortunes; it gives us a path to escape from our circumstances of misfortunes and allow us to regain who we are. Your life may appear to be filled with doubts, clouded with uncertainties, but a light of hope lies ahead. We can overcome these disappoints by joining together. Each and every one of us needs to set goals achievable, big or small. Set ten minutes certain time of the day to focus on your goals. If your goals seem difficult to achieve, join support groups that will motivate you. Never complaint about noting; focus your energy on yourself and give self-credits. We are all heroes of life's journey. You may not have a metal around your neck to show how much you have accomplished, but your inspiration will encourage someone you are not aware of to pursue a bigger dream. The caravan of love opens our eyes to aim high for bigger dreams and a brighter outcome. The caravan of love will erase our minds that are filled with doubts reopens our sense of self clouded with uncertainty and brings about positive self-esteems. We will not give up on anyone whether they are depressed or not aware of their own self-image.

There is a model of care for the caravan of love that I believe can be used to achieve obtainable goals. We have to focus on: Identification of the Problem, develop conflict resolution, review modifications approaches, to help develop resolution that will combat this problem. This includes educating the communities about the H.I.V virus and informs the people how this virus is transmitted and the illness it produces. This model can achieve great accomplishments if the people initiating and making the necessary adjustment will show empathy, be supportive, caring and compassionate to the sick. We do not know when we might be in a position where the help of another person is needed, so if we should put ourselves in the position of the other person for awhile, it will give us a sense of what these people are going through. We should not be judgmental of others because of the position they are in; we need to be supportive of our fellow human being. Giving care to someone who is at a stage of total dependence or need assistant from others, is wonderful; doing this makes the person feel wanted and love. Enriching our surrounding with these qualities enables the sick to have more dignity and respect for themselves. A model such as this one helps to ensure mobility, and improves positive outcomes for the sick. There should be no debate over this model; it is here to enforce good treatments, alleviate oversights, and to bring respect and dignity to us all; not only the sick. There are many options, but one choice remains: limit the spread of the HIV/AIDS virus.

True measures of a fellow human being is to rise to the occasion with outstretch arms willing to help another. We cannot afford to submit to failure; time matters. There need to be return of integrity to the people suffering from this deadly disease. We cannot continue to abide by a system that is not working; we have to embrace change of new approaches. We must realize that if the current system of helping people suffering from this disease is not fixed right away, then it comes harder to hold together. South Africa, though you are going through a dark day, we can find a ray of light shining through. Take advantage of the opportunity to make a change. It is a fact of life that things will be better with hard work.

It is now over thirty years since this disease the HIV/AIDS epidemic has made its initial impact. We have to consider the age range of people that cannot be ignored; not only for the HIV/AIDS epidemic, but for other sexual transmitted diseases. At the beginning of this crisis, we had people that were sexually active into their eighties. Now thirty years later, we have to look at an age range from teenagers to people in their eighties. We have young people who are sexually active, as well as the older population who were young when this disease was discovered. We also need to communicate the devastated emotional break down living with this disease causes upon an individual as well as their communities.

We have learned that HIV is a virus that attacks white blood cells that call helper T cells (CD4). These cells are part of the immune system that helps fight against bacteria that attacks the body. This virus makes the body vulnerable not being able to fight against infection. AIDS is a late stage of HIV infection; at this stage lot of damages have been done to the immune system. The HIV virus is acquired through exchange of body fluid from an infected person via blood, semen, breast milk or vaginal fluids. You are vulnerable if you engage in having multiple sexual partners, having sexual intercourse with a high risk behavior, born to an HIV infected mother, men who have sex with men, needle drug users, a health care worker being exposed to body fluids or being raped. I encourage regular doctor check up for those who are in a high risk group or someone with a suspected unfaithful sexual partner. Prevention include but are not limited to the following: abstinence, males use condoms, female purchase condoms to be used, talk to your partner about being faithful, do not have multiple sexual partners, do not share needles, and parents talk to your children about STD's.

Although global commitment to control the (HIV/AIDS pandemic has increased significantly in recent years, the virus continues to spread with alarming and increasing speed. No one country is free from this disease. With the increase spread of this disease globally, some countries have risen to the call for help from their people; others have logged behind and have allowed this disease to overwhelm their healthcare infrastructure. We can take a look at countries with low percentage of this disease base on their proactive approach and learn from them. This disease will not go away, but we can reduce it spread. We do this by being open and educate the public. Provide health care and medications for the infected. Open testing sites for people to go and check if they are infected. Have a network available to support the infected.

We are approaching the ending of this book; I ensure you, the trip has ended, but the journey continues. Traveling on the caravan of love has been a wonderful experience for me and I hope it was the same for you. Have you learn something on this journey? Will you encourage someone to join you on this journey? I have learned that nothing in life is guaranteed, but with strong determination to make this world a better place, by us continuing to focus on short and long term goals that will help build a great foundation of love and forgiveness. I hope I was successful in encouraging you to join me on the caravan of love. I cannot put a number to this measure; success is not measured by number, but by persistence determination to make a difference. I believe we are successful in convincing many to join in on the caravan of love, educating those who took this disease as a minor issue, even convincing some politician that the HIV virus is real, and most of all bringing comfort to the hearts of those who felt they weren't important because they are HIV positive.

We have come together on this journey bounded by faith to help those that are less fortunate than ourselves. We are not perfect! Yet we are called to participate in a mission directed to helping those that are physically ill, emotionally ill, and spiritually ill, those that are at a financial disadvantage state and others who need help and education. Our mission is to adhere to the belief that as human beings we can be better than our ancestors. We have come to understand on this mission that you and I are new leaders that will bring about enlightenment to the oppressed, restoration to the sick and peace to the dying. Our journey has taught us much about ourselves as well as others around us suffering from this deadly disease. We have learned to use our inner strength to give hope and to open the eyes of those who believed that sickness was the end that loosing a love one to AIDS was the end and that being infected with this HIV virus was the end.

We cannot forget the hard works of people around the communities that join in to help. Caregivers support is always needed whether the person is a mother, a father, grandparent, an extended family member, a friend or a good neighbor to the sick person. It is emotionally and psychologically delicate when it comes to asking for help for a sick person, especially when it comes upon being diagnose with HIV/AIDS. Most times people are so ashamed of letting anyone know that they are sick from such a disease because of the potential stigmatism that may follow. The person taken care of some diagnose with HIV/AIDS sometimes has to limit themselves from getting help that are available. This state of isolation sometimes leads to the caregiver becoming stressed and emotionally drained. In some rare cases, the sick person does not share with the caregiver the true causes of his or her sickness because of the shame it brings. Caregivers, you belong to a large community that is often times not known. You have stood in the gap for a love one who is unable to do for themselves, things they use to do for their selves. You may not be seen or recognized for your hard work, but help is on the way.

In a world where much wrong answers have not figured out as yet, we have done quite well on our journey. We found WMDD's. a generation waiting for outside help, advocates waiting to assist the needy, leaders proven to be courageous, reducing the barriers to HIV/AIDS education, exposing raping of young girls, eliminating pointing of fingers, gender inequalities where females are taken advantage of physically, emotionally and spiritually. This is a global crisis where no nation has an excuse not to join in and support the cry for help. We have figured out how to use our inner strength to give hope and open the eyes of those who believed that sickness was the end, listen to the cries for help, open our hearts to someone who has lost hope, and provide guidance so that people can identify their strength instead of allowing fear to be their primary source of hope. We need to turn to each other and not against one another. We need to over look policies of indifferences and focus more on the greater good of humanity. We must be tough enough to be advocating for the rights of those who cannot defend themselves; a little girl raped because she is a virgins, because it is believed that such an act can cure a male who is HIV positive.

We must be compassionate enough to allow the weak to cry on our shoulders, listen to the small voice of someone who was once an educator in their community. We should never be afraid to extend our arms around the shoulders of someone that words cannot comfort. We have learned to extend a hand without pointing a finger. I remember the staffs I met at the Hlabisa Hospital; continue to care for those babies left alone. The seven women and two men that travel from house to house to seek about children whose parents are dead, I thank you. The two men who open a canteen to feed children whose parents are too sick to cook and to send meals home for the sick parents, I am on my way back to share a receipt with you. Workers at the Africa Centre in Metubatuba, thank you for your hospitality. Doctor Hlengwa, I am on my way back to South Africa, it won't be this long ever.

Leaving South Africa was very sad for me. I felt as if I was leaving a dear friend who meant the world to me. For the short time I have spent there, you have captured my soul and set my mind on coming back. I have not forgotten you and I will never turn my back on you. To ease the pain I felt in my heart leaving you and to dry up the tears from my eyes, I comforted myself with the words of Bob Marley returning back home to America, "Waiting In Vain." South Africa, I know you do not want to wait in vain for my return. Now here I am. The words of Bob Marley:

From the very first time I blessed my eyes on you, South Africa!
My heart says "follow through"
It's my love that you're running to.

As much as I was so sad leaving South Africa, I was jamming, singing songs of restoration and freedom. I know there are lots of griefs and sufferings in South Africa, but sometime all that is needed, is for someone going through difficult times to hear that help is on the way. The caravan of love will not fail you; you have travel on this adventure to bring comfort to those who are suffering from this deadly disease. A simple smile can make a big difference in the life of someone going through difficult time; smile at someone less fortunate than you are. Smiling is contagious; this will allow someone to know that better days are ahead. We must learn to work together, knowing that we cannot survive without each other. Remember, this is not the end. There is no end to this book. You are the next chapter. Share it with someone, as we vow to make this world a better place to live. The caravan of love is our anchor. Despite arrays of setbacks and instabilities, we remain committed, our priorities is to maintain access to those who are sick and to educate those who are not about STD's. Vision without resources to me is a fantasy; you are our greatest assets in spreading this word. I stand by you to let you know that we can reduce the spread of the HIV virus.

Love is calling us to a higher place where there are no boundaries or traces of despair. Don't face the battle of life alone, embrace life one day at a time. The HIV crisis has been on going over many years. We have to encourage more responsibility, reduce false perceptions, impart realistic goals, and avoid discriminating against someone who has this virus. We must encourage individual responsibility, not to just hear, but to engage in reducing the spread of this disease. We have to work hard to achieve these goals; we cannot take shortcuts. Your sacrifices have rescued me. Your love has strengthened my weakened knees. Now I can run to a place where I can comfort and satisfied that emptiness deep within me. I no longer felt alone in my walk. The things that use to bother me are now small. I go to sleep hoping and expecting a better tomorrow. I do listen to the people around me, but

I am now satisfied with the little person deep inside. I do cry, but now not as often like before. On the caravan of love you have taken me up and down, forward and backward; you are the wave of the sea. I do not know where you get your energy, but in your presence, you fill my ears with music of love. You are my comforter, my protector.

At present, you may not see or know where you are going, but time will take us to our destiny. You have captured me and surround me with your love. Don't look back; we are moving ahead on this long journey. We are joining together, to journey to the end. With unity and determination of purpose we will achieve whatever goals set ahead of us. Some cannot measure success individually, but we can. Both individually and collectively we have done well and we still have a long way to go. Don't continue to be hostage of the pass; how quickly some of us forgot about the world we lived in a few years ago. Remember. Stand up for service, stand up for humanity, stand up for the less fortunate, and give of yourself. Now is the time to take a stand; stand up and join the caravan of love; travel in our BMW (Best Made Wagon). This will be a new beginning for many; I encourage you to forgive yourself of the past. Don't try to go back and fix failures of lost moments, use this energy to make a brighter future.

The long ongoing nightmare is coming to an end through educating the public, helping the sick, comforting the suffering, encouraging the fainted hearts, reminding the nay-Sayers that they are also vulnerable and informing the younger generations that they are at risk if they don't take universal precautions against these sexually transmitted diseases. Don't feel alone and neglected. Our battle plan did not become shattered after our first journey into heart land of this bottle. Often times battle plans become unscrambled after the start of a war, ours has not, instead it has become stronger. Looking back, his has been a true journey of faith. When you have the power to fix it, don't sweat it; live happy and let God take care of impossibilities. Feed your body soul and spirit with freedom, releasing opportunities in motion for a better future.

Remember I told you not long ago that we are always surrounded by light whether day or night. On this journey, there is something else I need to share with you. If the days or nights continue to be dark around us, there is light within us that will never go dim. You and I possess the ability to shine lights on some of the darkest moments in life. Let me remind you, as human beings, we are not perfect, yet call to be better than yesterday. You and I can release ourselves of weighty burdens by learning to forgive. The most important person we have to forgive first is ourselves; we have to learn to forgive ourselves before we can forgive others. With this ability, we can release ourselves of unfounded burdens and free others of theirs. Before a cure can be discovered for these sexually transmitted diseases, we can learn to forgive ourselves of mistakes made or the unpleasant nature of someone taking advantage of us. You did not know that you would become infected with a life-long disease by sharing your love with someone you trusted and felt safe with. If you were taken advantage of for whatever reasons, don't blame yourself. Saturate your minds and hearts with love. Burry bad memories where they can never be resurrected to haunt us again; and if they should ever come to our thoughts, don't try anything to get rid of them. Let them disappear on their own; after awhile they will discover that you or no longer afraid of them anymore. Excuses will keep us bounded, but when we can release ourselves by learning to forgive, go ahead and forgive. Forgiveness is the essence of restoring our innocent to a level where we will not be burden, but will be able to fly high above life's negative circumstances.

Now that you found out that you are HIV positive, I encourage you to take your antiretroviral medications as prescribed by your doctor. Furthermore, please don't forget to forgive yourself for becoming HIV positive. You have to first forgive yourself before trying to move on; remember love does not condones sadness, it only endures it. This will be part of accepting the responsibility for what happen. Now you might have had nothing to do with you acquiring the HIV virus, however, you have to relive yourself of this misfortune. Forgiving is a conscious and willing act on the part of one person to release bad thoughts about another person for doing something bad to them. It can be done passively or letting another person know how they offended you. Either way, you will have allowed yourself to be free from any revengeful thoughts. In the long run, you have allowed bad thoughts about another person to be discontinued. I encourage you to move on by encouraging pleasant thoughts about yourself and others.

In the early stage of the HIV/AIDS epidemic, people use to look at someone infected with the HIV/AIDS disease and made unwelcoming comments about them simple because of how the disease presented itself: looking malnourished, under weight, weak, having frequent diarrhea and lung diseases. A few years later after the discovery of antiretroviral drugs which lower the HIV virus load, people who were HIV positive were not looking like they did few years before the discovery of these medications. Now some people who know they are HIV positive were intentionally sleeping with other, having unprotected sex without sharing that they are HIV positive. Often times we find people to be inconsiderate to each other. During the early onset of this disease, people treated those infected with this disease inhumanely. Today when so much is known about this virus, we have people knowing that they are HIV positive, yet they intentionally infect others. We need to learn to love each other and be an advocate of forgiveness.

The journey on the caravan of love has not ended; it continues to pass through some of the most remote areas and well known cities on the face of the earth. Like the rush of a cold wintry wind on the face, you will be awaken on this journey and you will travel across this globe, awaken the sleepy and open the eyes of those failed to see that love can cure and set free a world destine for peace and freedom. This is our moment for all eyes to see. You cannot escape or hide from the need to care for those infected with this disease. Human optimism brings about changes for the improvement of our lives and a mission to help those in need. On this long journey, we have seen more of ourselves, than others. Honestly, progress has not come fast enough for many, yet we are fortunate to be here fighting for the good of humanity. We are confronting these challenges together. Unfortunately, despite the rapid spread of the HIV/AIDS epidemic, many countries have failed to set bench marks to help curb this disease. We talking and writing about the HIV/AIDS epidemic, to helps bring attention to this disease. Awhile back I shared with you the purpose of the sun and moon. There is something else I need to share with you. We all have events in our lives that appear to be unfair. Ever so often there are alignments between the sun and moon that is called an eclipse. This is when the sun and moon are equally aligned, and little to no sun light can be seen. Sometimes it appears as if we cannot escape from the down falls of life. Remember, although there appears to be no light coming from the sun, the sun is still shining. Be patient, in a short moment, sun light will reappears, displaying one of the most beautiful displays known to man; an eclipse. Progress does not unfold passively, or too aggressively, but through hard work and strong determination. Along the way you have been my unseen guest; a quiet listener, a comforter, sometimes angry, sometimes happy. I thank you. We are on the front line of this journey with strong determinations to reach across many fronts. Hope of a brighter beginning begins with us.

www.ingramcontent.com/pod-product-compliance
Lightning Source LLC
Chambersburg PA
CBHW020442290526
45785CB00002B/970